SACRAMENTO PUBLIC LIBRARY

SA

D0056400

FREE REFILLS

FREE REFILLS

A Doctor Confronts His Addiction

PETER GRINSPOON, M.D.

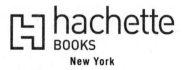

hachette
BOOKS
New York

Names and identifying characteristics have been changed including those of all of the author's patients, those he encountered in treatment, and most of the institutions that treated him.

Copyright © 2016 by Peter Grinspoon

All rights reserved. In accordance with the U.S. Copyright Act of 1976, the scanning, uploading, and electronic sharing of any part of this book without the permission of the publisher constitutes unlawful piracy and theft of the author's intellectual property. If you would like to use material from the book (other than for review purposes), prior written permission must be obtained by contacting the publisher at permissions@hbgusa.com. Thank you for your support of the author's rights.

Hachette Books
Hachette Book Group
1290 Avenue of the Americas
New York, NY 10104

www.HachetteBookGroup.com

Printed in the United States of America

RRD-C

First edition: February 2016
10 9 8 7 6 5 4 3 2 1

Hachette Books is a division of Hachette Book Group, Inc.

The publisher is not responsible for websites (or their content) that are not owned by the publisher.

Library of Congress Cataloging-in-Publication Data

Names: Grinspoon, Peter.
Title: Free refills : a doctor confronts his addiction / Peter Grinspoon, M.D.
Description: New York : Hachette Books, 2016.
Identifiers: LCCN 2015039428 | ISBN 9780316382700 (hardback) | ISBN 9781478960942 (audio download) | ISBN 9780316382687 (ebook)
Subjects: LCSH: Grinspoon, Peter—Health. | Physicians—Drug use—United States. | Physicians—United States—Biography. | BISAC: BIOGRAPHY & AUTOBIOGRAPHY / Medical. | BIOGRAPHY & AUTOBIOGRAPHY / Personal Memoirs.
Classification: LCC R154.G75 A3 2013 | DDC 610.92—dc23 LC record available at http://lccn.loc.gov/2015039428

For Lizzi.
Love you more.

How indeed could he hope to find himself, to begin again when, somewhere, perhaps, in one of those lost or broken bottles, in one of those glasses, lay, forever, the solitary clue to his identity?

—*Malcolm Lowry*, Under the Volcano

And what could a child know of the darkness of God's plan?

—*Cormac McCarthy*, Suttree

PART ONE

Free Refills

It was a frigid winter day in February 2005, when two officers—one from the state police, one from the Drug Enforcement Agency—arrived at my office and sat waiting amid the spellbinding view of the neighboring arboretum and the friendly clutter of charts, papers, stethoscopes, medical books, discarded coffee cups, and pharmaceutical samples.

At the time, I was scurrying back from a noon lecture on cholesterol management, in order to resume office hours. My attention was focused on the first patients I was soon to examine, an elderly Jewish couple plagued with anxiety and hemorrhoids, when, stethoscope in pocket and monogrammed white coat fluttering, I stopped dead still in the center of my office. My momentum was arrested by the concentrated accusatory gaze of the law enforcement authorities.

Unlike the patients in the packed waiting room, these officers didn't have the uncomfortable and deferential "I'm waiting for my prostate exam" look. Rather, their demeanor more resembled that of famished carnivores.

Far from famished, Rufus, the police officer, was morbidly obese, pasty, and spoke with a thick Boston accent. Bruno, the DEA agent, was thin, sarcastic, and fake friendly. He seemed as if he wanted to put his feet on my desk. (Why certainly, your Federalness. Go right ahead.)

Reflexively, I started hedging, stalling for time, trying to create some understandable context for their presence in my office. "My wife, H., gave me your business card yesterday, and I've been meaning to call you. I'm really glad that you are here, and that—" Bruno waved his hands dismissively and interrupted me with, "Doc, cut the crap already. We know you've been writing bad scrips."

Bruno and Rufus weren't here to arrest me and drag me outside in front of my staff or, worse, my patients, bumping my head against the top of their cruiser as they stuffed me into the backseat. They didn't read me my Miranda rights or pull out guns. They didn't yell, "Freeze, and put your hands up!" They didn't handcuff me, shock me with Tasers, club me with riot sticks, or detonate any canisters of tear gas in my office. They didn't hunker down behind my desk and radio in for reinforcements, bawling into their handsets, "All units, we've got a doctor here who is taking drugs!"

Instead, seemingly with relish, they informed me that I was to be charged with three felony counts of fraudulently obtaining a controlled substance. They had evidence that I had written prescriptions for the powerful narcotic Vicodin in the name of a former nanny, who had long since returned home to New Zealand, and that I had been picking them up from the pharmacy for my own use. They were tipped off by an astute pharmacist at CVS.

They say the universe is still gradually expanding, but at that moment, my universe started collapsing, even imploding, like a balloon stuck with a pin. Just minutes earlier, I was blithely sipping on gourmet coffee and chomping down doughnuts that some drug rep had dropped off (trying to push, no doubt, a cholesterol-lowering drug) while daydreaming through some lunchtime lecture. I had the expectation of a moderately hectic but lucrative afternoon examining grateful patients, and then returning home to see my kids.

Suddenly I was facing serious legal and career uncertainty, and was feeling awash in guilt and confusion. I had dealt with handcuffs during the tumultuous years I worked for Greenpeace, and knew that they were child's play compared to what my wife, H., was going to do to me when she learned of these charges. I'd take a Taser any day. And what about my kids? Were they going to be allowed to visit me in the penitentiary, waving at me through dirty plastic and speaking to me through a buzzing telephone connection?

At that point, I decided that I had had enough drama for one day, so I tried to politely signal to Bruno and Rufus that office hours were over. Doctors are excellent at dismissing people. We stand up, indicate toward the door with body language, ruffle some papers, and say something pithy about how we hope their fungus, or whatever is ailing them, feels better soon.

Unfortunately, Bruno and Rufus were just warming up. They pressured me with not-so-veiled threats. "Doc, we're here just trying to get you the help you need. If you tell us what we need to know, we don't have to blab to the other docs here and to your patients." They were threatening to expose me if I didn't sing, and to leave no stone unturned.

"Who else has been writing scrips for you? What other docs? Give us names. How else do you get pills? Buy them on the streets? Do you shoot up? Snort? Sell pills on the side? What other drugs do you use? Weed? Coke? Heroin? Angel dust?"

Under duress, my mind started wandering. I couldn't help thinking, "Since when do doctors do angel dust? Get with the times."

Once this line of questioning dried up, they tried a different tactic. "Doc, if your wife is popping these pills, you will never get out of this." They had the pleasure of meeting her the day before. According to the police report,

On 2/16/2005 at approximately 3:30 p.m. S/A XXXXX and TFO XXXXX went to —— Street, _____, MA and were met by H. who later identified herself as the wife of Peter Grinspoon, M.D. H. appeared nervous and agitated and refused to speak to S/A XXXXX and TFO XXXXX and further asked that they return with a uniformed officer if they wanted to speak to her. At approximately 5:00 p.m. S/A XXXXX and TFO XXXXX returned to the previously stated address accompanied by Boston Police Patrolman

Andrew XXXXX. At this time, H. had a normal demeanor and agreed to speak with the officers. H. was asked if she knew R—— S—— and she responded that she has employed Ms. S—— as an au pair through International Au Pair. H. further said Ms. S—— left the U.S. in January 2004 and returned to New Zealand. At this time the interview was terminated.

Oh yeah. H. mentioned that the police came by. Really bizarre pillow talk. "Honey, the police stopped by today to ask about our former nanny." I should have made a run for it. Possibly, just possibly, I could have made it over the Canadian border and spared myself the misery of the next few years. Good-bye wife. Good-bye children. Good-bye career as a primary care doctor.

I answered that no, thanks for your concern, but unfortunately, my wife doesn't take prescription painkillers, and I was the one who had a problem.

Why would I admit that to them? What would I say next? I prided myself on being a cunning drugstore cowboy, but this situation was feeling increasingly out of control, like a bad episode of *Law & Order*. I started to grasp that Bruno and Rufus had a broader agenda than just "getting me the help I need." They wanted to nail me. They were somehow getting me to divulge things that should be kept private, to fill in the details for them, and to hoist myself on my own petard. The police report further reads,

At this time S/A XXXXX told GRINSPOON that he had been prescribing hydrocodone in the name of P—— X—— and picking up the prescriptions. GRINSPOON said he had written eight prescriptions for hydrocodone with refills and stated half had been for him and half were for P—— X——. S/A XXXXX and TFO XXXXX further asked GRINSPOON weren't all the prescriptions for him? GRINSPOON replied that from 8/17/2004 through to 2/15/2005 all controlled substances written for P—— X—— by him were used by him.

At that point, I suggested that I get a lawyer. This was like pulling the final control rod out of the Fukushima nuclear reactor. Bruno and Rufus became bullying and hostile. "Doc, we could arrest you right now, cuff you, drag you out in front of your staff." I summoned my inner donkey, and the interview ended in a Mexican standoff. They instructed me to report to police headquarters at 8:00 a.m. the next morning to be booked and fingerprinted, and left in a huff. Have a nice day. Thanks for stopping by.

I was born at the Boston Lying-In Hospital, in the heart of Harvard Medical School, so that the pressure for me to become a doctor at Harvard could be inhaled with my first breath. My twin brother, Martin, born four minutes earlier, was allowed to go home several days before I did, because he hogged most of the food in utero and I was underweight coming out of the womb, weighing in at just over five pounds.

Being so scrawny, I was relegated to the preemie nursery for the better part of a week. Had we been able to speak, he would have said, "See you later, sucker. Now I get first pick of crib space and Binkies at home." I would have replied, "You shameless pig! Just wait until I can crawl. I'll make you pay!"

I've often wondered if they could have switched us in the hospital. Back then, in 1966, they weren't as uptight about identity bracelets on newborns. That would mean that I am him and he is me. Hey, Bruno, hey, Rufus. You incompetent bullies, you've arrested the wrong guy.

Assuming we weren't switched, why did I become an addict and he didn't? Were our lives really so different? Was it the trauma and influence of being stuck in the preemie nursery that set me on the wrong path from day one? Did I encounter some perinatal pre–gang members who corrupted me? Maybe someone said, "Gaa gaaa gooo goooo" ("Yo, homey, let's go smoke a spleef"). After all, the Boston Lying-In Hospital was in a bad part of town. It was located in Boston's notorious Mission Hill neighborhood.

Or maybe it was bad karma? Perhaps in a previous life I was a marauding Visigoth, chewing on human skulls, and he was a peaceable man of the cloth. Was it a random assortment of genes? Maybe I am just a victim of the law of averages.

Or did I lose some intrauterine game of rock, paper, scissors over who had to shoulder the family mantle of becoming a doctor, with the stress and sleeplessness of this calling. By becoming a doctor, you can improve the health of thousands, but it's not necessarily good for your own health.

To this day, Martin asserts that all of my problems result from the immaturity associated with my being four minutes younger than him.

On the wall of my childhood home is a picture of me when I was two years old. I am staring straight into the camera as if startled by it, with wide blue eyes and fluffy brown hair. My finger is stuck into a crack in the stone wall I'm standing next to. A minute later I'll start to cry, when I can't get my finger out of the wall without twisting it. Most telling of all is the Harvard Medical diaper I'm wearing.

As soon as the fuzz left my office, I told my staff that I had a migraine and had them cancel my patients for the rest of the day. This was the second sick time I'd ever taken. I must have looked convincingly ill, because I was drenched in sweat and I was shaking from head to toe. My medical assistant expressed sympathy, which I felt I didn't deserve.

I promptly swallowed the eight oxycodone I had hidden in my bag in a bottle labeled ALLERGY MEDICINE. In case of emergency, break glass and swallow pills. I was desperately hoping this oxycodone would cause what I warn patients about: sedation, amnesia, euphoria, and a false sense of well-being. I didn't think I could possibly get into more trouble, though, in retrospect, a DUI would have been the straw that broke the camel's back.

With extra care, I creeped my car out of the parking lot and, granny-like, navigated the brief drive back to my home. I remember a vivid escape fantasy where I just kept driving and left all of this behind me. With my credit cards, how far could I get before anyone noticed I was missing? Would these criminal charges stop me at the border?

During this drive, I was having trouble piecing together how I ended up with two agents tracking snow, and criminal charges, into my office. How did I descend into the cunning mind frame of a common criminal? Last time I checked, I was a successful and empathic doctor. At the same time, a small part of me was feeling a Raskolnikov-like sense of relief, thinking, "Thank God this is going to end."

Parking the car with care, I glanced briefly at the closely set, shabby, but well-tended houses of our lower-middle-class blue-collar neighborhood, steeled myself, said a quiet good-bye to the life I knew, a life built on lies, said some sort of good-bye to myself, and walked into the vestibule of our comfortably furnished Victorian home.

Our house still smelled faintly like reefer from a private smoking session H. and I had had a few nights before. H. has red hair, a trim figure, and clear blue eyes. She is quick to smile but quicker to anger. On the occasional times we smoked together, H. became amorous, demanded chocolate, demanded sex, and then fell into a deep sleep. What more could a guy ask for? Legalize it!

At all other times, I was lonely, and I clutched at any crumb of tenderness she would toss my way. I was desperate for these rare bonding moments, because I was increasingly alienated from my marriage. The night after our wedding, H. started talking in her sleep, vitriolic speeches criticizing me, as if we were in Salem's Lot and she were possessed by the undead. It gave me goosebumps and insomnia. Daytime wasn't much better.

In the living room, I was met by friendly commotion and bustle. "Daddy's home!" Anne, who was five years old and who has penetrating blue eyes, and Milo, who was four, with dirty-blond hair, boisterous and fun-loving, raced each other to get to me first and hug my legs, elbowing each other out of the way. They are almost "Irish twins," a mere fourteen months apart in age.

H. greeted me as if nothing were amiss, though I could tell she was suspicious that I was home early. That wasn't my role. I was supposed to be earning.

I switched into robot mode and completed what was required of me for the rest of the day. Something about this unconditional love from my kids made me feel like an imposter, and I had a dark premonition that I was going to be seeing less of them.

Later, when the children were asleep, and H. and I retired to our cozy double bed, I wasn't sure how to broach the day's events. "Hi, honey, the police were in my office today and I've ruined our life." No, that didn't sound right. "Hi, honey, you look beautiful and, by the way, I might be going to prison and you might have to work full time." No better.

H. can become furious about a dish being left in the sink, or an unmade bed. So, naturally, I was not enthusiastic about mentioning the fact that criminal charges were impending and that it wouldn't be clear for quite a while whether my medical license would be returned to me during this lifetime. I dove in and gave an honest and thorough description of what had transpired.

This conversation didn't go well.

"You fucking asshole. You asshole. I've been telling you, you're a drug addict, and now you have ruined our lives."

"Look, H., I'm really sick and I need help. I feel really bad about this."

What else could I say? Technically, I was guilty as charged, though I was hoping for some warmth and compassion, and I felt hurt and betrayed by her reaction.

Granted, H. had suffered the fallout of my steady descent into uncontrolled pill-popping over the last six years. When I told her this news, I wasn't expecting praise or congratulations. I wasn't expecting her to stand up and applaud, or to offer sexual favors, or to nominate me for husband of the year. But after seven years of marriage, I did hope for at least some sympathy and nurturing. Some sense of "I'm here for you; we'll get through this together." Or at least an acknowledgment of how sick and miserable I was and how painful my current circumstances were. No dice.

Later, burrowed into my new habitat, the downstairs sofa, whose pillows didn't quite connect together in a way that permitted sleep without back pain, and whose dusty covers triggered my allergies, I started formulating some questions to myself. How exactly did I get caught? I had committed hundreds of illegal acts over the last few years; it wasn't clear to me which ones had led to the criminal charges. Am I really caught, or can I talk my way out of this? Am I possibly going to jail? Is this going to be on the front page of the *Boston Globe*? Will I ever practice medicine again? What is wrong with me anyway? All in all, it was a long night on the sofa.

Upon awakening, I Googled the address of the police station I had to report to. Canceling work in order to avoid being arrested at my office was as good an excuse as any, so I left a message on my secretary's voice mail, claiming ill health and letting her know that I wouldn't be coming in to work that day. (Or ever again?) I felt bad about this because, short of being hospitalized once for viral meningitis, I hadn't missed a day on the job, stoically working despite colds, stomach flus, and headaches. Doctors are mostly expected to continue working no matter how they are feeling, which is part of the problem.

At five in the morning, hopelessly awake and eager to avoid another interaction with H., I skulked into the bedroom to get my clothes for the day and, unable to face Annie or Milo either, I left the house, bought acidic, burnt coffee at 7-Eleven, mooned around for a while, and then, at daybreak, started driving toward the police station on South Boston's waterfront.

On the way, I passed the clinic in "Southie" where I trained as a medical student. It was where I had my first, fumbling experiences interviewing patients and listening to their insides. Passing that health center reminded me of this earlier phase of my life, when I was an eager, enthusiastic medical student with a universe of opportunity in front of me, chomping at the bit to learn as much as possible and to start trying to heal people.

The police station was dingy, dilapidated, and sparsely populated. It was just waking up for the day, and I was its first client. It was all so drab, I felt as if I were in a black-and-white film.

Rufus was waiting for me when I arrived and, for all his look of studied nonchalance, booking a doctor was clearly out of the ordinary for him, a highlight in a career that I imagined was otherwise spent dealing with low-level thugs and traffic violations. Businesslike, condescending, and without the warmth or feigned concern he showed the day before, he guided me into the special area, behind the large front counter, where a computerized fingerprinting apparatus was set up. "Sit down and stick your hands out." (I guess that's better than "Bend over.")

I hadn't anticipated that this process would be computerized, which meant that my fingerprints would never be lost and that I would be tagged for life. I wondered if my twin brother had the same fingerprints. With every molecule of his three-hundred-plus-pound bulk, Rufus squashed the fingers of my right hand onto the glass screen, attempting to push my hand through the table. As my fingers started burning, I began to grasp more fully the seriousness of my predicament.

Rufus then told me about the three charges being filed against me, identical to one another, all felonies, which read as follows:

Criminal Complaint: 94C/33/C Drug, Obtain by Fraud. On 1/29/2005 did knowingly or intentionally acquire or obtain possession of a controlled substance by means of forgery, fraud, deception or subterfuge, in violation of G. L. c.94C (PENALTY: state prison not more than 4 years; or house of correction not more than 2 1/2 years; or not more than $20,000 fine; or both such imprisonment and fine).

I was told to report to the West Roxbury courthouse on a date to be provided, not more than ten days hence.

Rufus watched me like a hawk as I drove away. Perhaps he fantasized that I'd commit a moving violation and that he could then take some more fingerprints, on my left hand, which still had intact nerves and blood vessels. Carefully dodging the wired and aggressive Boston drivers, I drove home slowly in order to have some time to internalize what had just happened. With no audience to impress, I started shaking like a leaf.

That night, when the kids were in bed, I wanted to give H. a sanitized version of the day's events, but things were so bad, and I was so worn down, I had no choice but to be open and honest. In an icy, detached voice, H. said, "If you can't work as a doctor, you are going to work at Home Depot. If you are in legal trouble, your parents better pay our legal fees." Then she rolled over, with her back to me, and fell asleep. I trudged downstairs to the sofa.

Martin and I are now five, and we are following our older brothers, Danny, at age thirteen, and David, age eleven, on one of our earliest acts of familial ecoterrorism. This was a full seventeen years before I started working for Greenpeace.

Behind our childhood home is a seemingly endless expanse of woods, which Babson College, an up-and-coming business school, is trying to clear-cut so that they can demonstrate to their students how to turn a profit by destroying the environment. To us, this is clearly wrong, and we are intent on stopping it.

Our parents are not particularly intent on preventing us from stopping Babson, so they explain to us that there is a drainage system slowly siphoning the entire woods in preparation for clear-cutting and paving. All we have to do is dam up the shallow creek that runs behind our house, cause a flood, and delay the project, hopefully for years. This becomes our mission in life. We spend every free moment cementing stones with mud and sticks into increasingly elaborate dams, which were designed by Danny.

As afternoons floated by blissfully, working together on our dam in the sun and the mud and the gently trickling creek, I was unaware that Babson would succeed in paving much of this forest, and that my brother Danny was slowly dying. It was only much later that I understood about the wigs, the nausea, the mood changes in the other family members, and the sweet-smelling smoke.

Danny had always been an involved and affectionate older brother who wrestled with us and invented games for us to play. Maybe on some level he sensed he didn't have much time with us. He talked my parents into letting us paint the walls and ceiling of the closet in his room with black-light paints, so that we had a private room that glowed eerily under the black light we bought. This room was a private, magical space where, as kids, we were able to create our own world. (Or, as teenagers, get high.) We worshipped Danny like a Roman emperor.

We weren't old enough to notice that Danny was losing weight, or that he had lost his hair. I didn't even know that he wore a wig. Nor did we notice that, at times, he didn't quite seem his usual playful self.

With criminal charges filed, it was only a matter of time until the medical board yanked my license to practice.

Immediately upon leaving the police station, my first phone call was to set up an emergency meeting with Society to Help Physicians (SHP), an affiliate of the Medical Society of Massachusetts that helps physicians with depression, grief, drugs, alcohol, personality disorders, and disruptive behaviors. A hidden truth is that doctors crack under pressure like anyone else, and might even be more susceptible to depression and addiction. I was hoping SHP could provide cover. I felt I needed to keep working, because I had several thousand patients who were counting on me. I could even get sued for "abandonment" if I stopped treating my patients.

SHP provided a list of lawyers with specialty in the area of docs on drugs. Like the police, SHP told me that I didn't have a choice but to report to them at 8:00 a.m. the next day. This eight-in-the-morning thing was getting repetitive.

I had already made initial contact with SHP a couple of months earlier. I had been seeing an addiction counselor in response to an ugly threat by my regular psychiatrist to report me to the medical board as an "impaired physician." I was seeing this psychiatrist in order to treat depression and insomnia, which had plagued me since my teenage years.

My addiction counselor was named Ben. Ben tried to maintain a sense of personal gravitas despite wearing leather and biker boots, chain-smoking cigarettes, having long hair, and sporting a goatee. He could seem needy and insecure, and I felt like we spent most of our sessions focusing on his breakup instead of my problems. He had a reputation for being warm and fuzzy.

During our first meeting, Ben also threatened to report me to the medical board as an impaired physician unless I set up an appointment to meet with Dr. Stern at SHP within two weeks. So far, Ben seemed about as warm and fuzzy as a crocodile.

Dr. Stern's office was in a sterile, corporate office building, otherwise occupied by medically related Internet companies. It is contiguous with Fenway Park, which is a nightmarish place to drive to and park, especially if one doesn't share a special reverence for the Red Sox.

After I got past security and endured a short but nerve-racking wait, Dr. Stern lumbered in and brought me back to his office, which was the unapologetic den of an absentminded professor. It was cluttered with books, journals, articles, even some stale candy, which I was offered but was afraid to touch. The candy bowl itself was covered with dust and had a few imprinted marks where clients more desperate than I had succumbed to this invitation. Newly sober alcoholics tend to crave sugar.

Dr. Stern was a frumpy, lean, preachy, and seemingly sluggish man, with pasty skin and thinning blond hair. He was obviously very pious, which, right off the bat, allowed my atheistic eyes to invalidate him and the message he was trying to convey.

One of the central intellectual principles that had been ingrained in me since childhood was that religion, as Karl Marx said, is "the opiate of the people." In Dr. Stern's office, I silently and condescendingly marveled at this irony: This man was supposed to help me get off drugs, not substitute one for another. When he explained that, in his younger days, he had lost his medical license to drugs and had spent time behind bars, he started to rise in my estimation.

My goal was to appear cooperative but to reveal as little as possible. Dr. Stern and Ben knew each other from both being members of the small Boston addiction treatment community.

Dr. Stern had been tipped off by Ben that I was a bullshit artist. As they say, "You can't bullshit a bullshitter." He didn't fall for my evasions.

I was hoping to come across as an exemplar of abstemious rectitude, so as to stop this evaluation dead in its tracks. My addiction was fighting for its life. I took a deep breath and dove in. "I don't know why I'm here. Sometimes I smoke pot. So do lots of other people. Ideally, I shouldn't touch pills, but I get migraines. My doctor prescribes them. I also have insomnia, so my shrink gives me Klonapin. It's all legitimate, except for the pot, which is harmless and should be legal. What else would you like to know?"

Dr. Stern looked as if he had stepped on something unpleasant. "By using these pills, you have changed your brain chemistry forever. You are unable to control this." I retorted, "That's crap; you don't know anything about me. I can totally control this. Things are going great at work. This is much ado about nothing."

Dr. Stern specializes in this field and had seen the incarnation of what I was trying to do dozens of times before. "If you stop doing drugs, everything will be OK, but if you don't, your untreated addictions will inevitably lead to one of three places: jail, an institution, or death. You will lose your job and your medical license. You will soon find yourself in legal trouble as well as marital trouble. The wives of addicts can be unforgiving bitches. You are going to end up like David Arndt [a talented local surgeon who left a patient on the table in the middle of surgery to visit an ATM machine in order to pay for methamphetamine]. You need to sign one of our monitoring contracts and start with the drug testing immediately."

At that point, I still had the luxury to decline the services of SHP. I said something to the effect of "Thank you very much for your concern. We'll be in touch. It's been nice chatting with you. Good luck. Godspeed," and blithely sped out of his office toward my Percocet supply, thinking, "Wow, he was easy to fool."

At the time, I didn't know what a vast impact this humble, prescient man would have on my future.

Now, a mere two months later, with Bruno and Rufus appointed as my new guardian angels, with the medical board about to shit-can me, and with H. transformed into a fifty-megaton hydro-gen bomb, Dr. Stern's predictions were proving to be ruinously accurate.

If nothing else, I had become leery of Stern's prediction-making ability. I wondered if he could pick stocks.

Now, shortly after my arrest, tail between legs, the fear of a figurative God in me, I was forced back to Society to Help Physi-cians. I was not just there to meet with Dr. Stern, but to meet with the entire leadership of SHP. As I crossed the threshold, I didn't stop to consider what SHP would ask in return for their assistance, that they would impose a reverse Faustian bargain in which where they would hound me with drug tests until I got my soul back. Good luck with that.

SHP is housed in the ostentatious headquarters of the Medi-cal Society of Massachusetts. The building was conceived dur-ing an earlier age, when doctors were wealthy and important, not minions of the insurance and pharmaceutical companies. It is sar-castically referred to as the Taj Mahal because of its grandiose design.

Entering that beehive of successful and ambitious doctors, with my fingers still sore from the flattening they underwent at the hands of Rufus the day before, I felt adrift and unshaven. As a foil to my predicament, the doctors here were well dressed, confident, and moving purposefully. It appeared that they must all have happy families and unblemished careers. I couldn't have less in common with them.

SHP has a complex dual role, simultaneously advocating for physicians and policing them. Their monitoring contract requires weekly random urine drug screens, support group meetings, ther-apy, and abstention from all mood-altering chemicals, including alcohol. No mouthwash or NyQuil, both of which contain alco-hol. No OFF! or hand sanitizer, which are alcohol based. No rum cake. No poppy seeds, which show up as a narcotic on a drug screen, because heroin is derived from poppies.

The monitoring contract was binding for three to five years. Most ominously, it required a week-long inpatient evaluation at the Talbott Recovery Center in Atlanta, to determine whether I needed a longer stay in rehab. I was expecting a slap on the wrist, but this program had teeth sharp enough to make Jaws look like he was wearing dentures.

SHP pretended that my signing the contract was volitional, and it's true no one was physically forcing me to sign. There was no gun to my head and no thumbscrews (or thumb Rufuses). Though I knew, and they knew, and they knew that I knew, that without signing this contract I was sunk. My medical license would be revoked and I'd be defenseless against the felony charges I was facing.

In essence, I had lost the luxury of pondering, in an abstract sense, how drug screens might impinge upon my civil liberties. Signing this contract was the only way to signal that I was serious about getting help. The problem was that, if I signed, I would *have* to get help, which, at the time, I had no intention of doing.

Sitting alone, reading the proposed SHP monitoring contract, waiting for their nice but short and businesslike attorney to re-explain all of the restrictions on me, and all of the hoops I would have to jump through for the next several years, I wondered if I'd ever be able to practice medicine again.

True, at that moment I still had my license and my job, but I was waiting for the ax to fall. The medical board wouldn't let felony charges go unpunished. They are in perpetual "cover your ass" mode. Even if they wanted to be lenient, or understanding of addiction as a medical disease, they were hamstrung, because then they would be vulnerable to criticism if anything bad happened with any of my patients, even if it wasn't my fault. Their paranoid fantasy is an above-the-fold headline in the *Boston Globe*: MEDICAL BOARD ALLOWS DRUGGED-OUT DOCTOR TO KILL INNOCENT PATIENTS. LAWMAKERS CALL FOR INVESTIGATION.

Contemplating this contract, I felt my hard work to become a doctor—the sleepless nights, the endless studying, the high-pressure exams, and the $200,000 tuition—I felt all of this becoming insubstantial. I wondered who would provide for my children. I fantasized about having to return to my high school job at McDonald's, wearing a shabby, stained uniform, often poisoned by McNugget overdose, and getting yelled at by acne-ridden obese managers as I carried heavy, steaming buckets of grease to dump into the fetid dumpster behind the restaurant. If McDonald's now required a criminal background check, I wouldn't even get my old job back.

Out of options, fearful of the future, I signed their contract. They had succeeded in extracting a pound of drugged-out flesh. For my ID card, they took a photograph that looked like a mug shot, on a bad hair day, with bloodshot eyes and a bewildered, despairing expression. From now on, I was #1270. They gave me instructions about where to go for drug testing later that day and for my support group meeting that night.

Compounding my problems, despite a modest stockpile, I hadn't dared pop any pills since the eight Percocet following fun time with Bruno and Rufus. Molecule by molecule, my body degraded whatever narcotics were left in my system. Within twelve hours, I had started feeling as if I had the worst possible case of the flu, as well as a deep depression. I no longer felt comfortable in my skin, and I had stomach cramps and severe diarrhea. I felt awful by the time I set out to meet my new attorney, Solomon.

January 13, 1973, was an icy morning outside, and was seemingly a typical weekend morning, with David, Martin, and me cuddled up under our worn but cozy leopard-patterned blanket, watching Saturday morning cartoons. Danny wasn't with us, but we were accustomed to that, because he had been spending more time in the hospital. This was always spoken of in euphemisms. He was "away, getting better."

On this particular Saturday, my dad came down the stairs looking worn and grave. He made us turn off the television, a bad sign, and said that he needed to speak with us, an even worse sign. Usually this would mean that we had smashed or broken something in the house and were about to be punished, so he captivated our complete attention.

He announced, "Your brother Danny passed away last night." Despite the best efforts of the Dana-Farber Cancer Institute and the brightest Harvard doctors, after six years of fighting, all the available medications had slowly failed. (Today, children with acute lymphocytic leukemia have a 99 percent survival rate due to medical advances.) The last week of Danny's life was spent in a coma, with my dad at the bedside.

I didn't know how to respond to this announcement. I didn't feel as sad as I would have felt if I had any idea what it meant. I knew that "passing away" meant dying, and I knew that "dead" was a bad state, with something vaguely wrong or shameful associated with it. At that moment, seven years old, I didn't understand that I would never see Danny again.

But I knew enough to see that my dad was at the end of his rope, and to look sad and to act respectfully. I knew not to ask to turn the TV back on, despite my curiosity about what would happen next to Speed and Trixie. I knew enough not to try to yank the leopard-patterned blanket away from my brothers, or to give my twin a surreptitious kick, as I ordinarily might do.

Danny's illness affected my life from the moment I became aware of him being sick. At home, I could sense that something was very wrong; I just didn't know what. When you are seven, there is no perspective or context. You hear your parents talking about a broken car, a stain on a rug, or a brother in the hospital, and it's impossible to rank these in order of importance.

My attorney Solomon's office was next to Boston's South Station, in a huge, gleaming, corporate office building. Everything in the lobby seemed fake and sterile, even the plants. When I looked closely, I saw they were covered with dust, just like Dr. Stern's bowl of candy. I sensed a common theme. As I made my rounds of shame, I was greeted by dust.

When I tried to bend a leaf, I found it was made of unyielding plastic. This effort left a fingerprint in the dust, which would have helped Rufus, had he been on my trail. There was a waterfall in the lobby, splashing over black rocks, with dirty nickels and dimes on the bottom, and a few pieces of floating debris. Even though we were inside, I half expected pigeons to land and start pecking at crumbs.

On the thirty-fifth floor, the waiting room was staffed by tanned, fit, bleach blondes, who politely offered me coffee while I waited, and went back to reading *People* magazine. After a long wait, which communicated that my time wasn't as valuable as his, I was greeted by a tall Jewish man, who was immaculately dressed.

Solomon brought me down to his office, which was lined with musty law books that appeared as if they were there for effect and hadn't been read. No one can read that many books. Solomon sat behind a large mahogany desk. He also looked as if he had stepped on something unpleasant. I was beginning to get a complex.

In a sarcastic, distant tone of voice, looking paternal and displeased, he began: "To what do I owe the pleasure of your company? This isn't on the record, but tell me honestly and fully what you did and where things stand, and we'll see what we can do." I replied, "I'm in a lot of trouble with the law, and the medical board, and I need your help."

Solomon conveyed confidence and competence but was not particularly empathic. I felt like I was his meal ticket. As with most attorneys I had dealt with, I had the sense that he was being agreeable and polite only because I was paying him $400 per hour. Sort of like prostitution. If he had happened to be on the other side of this particular dispute, he wouldn't be sympathetic. He'd be ripping me to shreds.

Realizing that, at the very least, my friendliness toward patients was genuine and consistent made me proud to be a doctor, until I realized that I might not be one for much longer.

After bringing him up to speed, I asked him to summarize where we were. He said that the medical board tends to be conservative and is unpredictable, but if I complied perfectly with my Society to Help Physicians contract, I would have a chance of being able to continue to practice medicine, uninterrupted by a suspension. Otherwise, I could be sidelined for as long as several years, if not indefinitely.

He assured me that he'd take care of matters on his end, and that at some point, possibly sooner than later, things would be OK, under one nonnegotiable condition: "Don't, under any circumstances, no matter what happens, don't fail any of your drug tests." Piece of cake.

A few days after my interview with Solomon, we appeared together in court for my summons, during which I was formally charged with three felonies. On the way in, security confiscated the handheld voice recorder I had in my bag, which I had been using to record H. No one, not even my twin brother, fully believed me when I described the desperation of our current marital conditions, until they heard one word of the bone-chilling voice of anger. That was all it took. If there were a branch of Amnesty International that represented the rights of voice recorders, I would have been blacklisted.

One thinks of courthouses as august institutions, the cornerstones of our democracy, so I was shocked to find that everything was shabby: The uniforms of the guards were wrinkled, and the rug was dirty, with a nauseating pattern of barf-colored swirls. Of course there was dust. Paint was chipping from the walls. Scraggly plants, if alive at all, drooped from plastic hangers, as if they had heard the same hard-luck cases too many times. The windows were filthy, filtering gray light. Third-rate lawyers roamed the halls, herding sad or angry-looking people from place to place. Pictures of dead judges were hanging on the walls, attempting to look kindly and impartial but mostly looking dead. Musty smells, white noise, murmurs, and coughs. The wooden benches were excruciating, direct descendants of the Spanish Inquisition, designed to injure the tailbone. The bailiff circulated, jocular yet menacing, threatening people for using cell phones, talking, or, God forbid, reading.

The bailiff bellowed "All rise," and en masse we stood up as the judge entered. She was a stern-looking gray-haired woman with intelligent eyes and a dignified demeanor. I wondered how such a distinguished-looking judge had ended up at such a dilapidated courthouse. Maybe she was an underachiever, or struggled with alcoholism. She sat down at her dais, flanked by flags, with the round seal of ye olde commonwealth of Massachusetts as the backdrop.

Most of the other cases that were heard involved petty thefts and domestic disputes. I was too preoccupied to pay attention, unless there was some lurid reference to sex or violence.

I sensed the atmosphere in the courthouse change when they called my name. Probably because they called me Dr. So-and-so instead of Mr. So-and-so. To a bored courtroom, this was more attention-grabbing than sex and violence. So much for staying anonymous. Were any of my patients here?

I walked up to the stand, and the charges against me were read out loud. Three felonies. To the court officers, I was both doctor and felon, so I was treated with a confusing amalgam of ingrained respect for my profession and habitual disdain for the low-life scumbags that are paraded through. This was unsettling, because I was used to the former, not the latter.

The judge, after conferring with both Solomon and the prosecuting attorney, set a date a few months later when my legal disposition would be decided, and then halted the courtroom proceedings, locked her forceful gaze on me, and, with a cold professionalism that betrayed genuine humanity underneath, simply said, "Good luck with your recovery, Doctor." This was enough to momentarily break the spell of hopelessness that I was under, and I looked up from staring at the floor to thank her.

Upon leaving, I actually did bump into one of my patients who works as a constable, complete with a concealed weapon, which I had noticed strapped to his ankle during a physical exam. I felt compelled to make up an excuse to explain my presence in his stomping ground. I said I was "weighing in on a patient's disposition," whatever that meant. I actually had an appointment with him the next morning. "See ya tomorrow, Doc." For the moment, I still had my medical license and the respect of my patients.

At the time of my brother Danny's illness, there were no effective treatments for the nausea and weight loss associated with chemotherapy. My parents begrudgingly allowed him to try cannabis. According to the story that I've heard my father tell dozens of times on TV and in print as well as in person, Danny found that, after a few puffs, he could hold food down soon after the chemo sessions. He was even hungry.

I have a vague memory, from when I was just five or six, of our parents going out, leaving Danny, David, Martin, and me to our own devices. We had a live-in "mother's helper" who must have also been gone, or might have been asleep upstairs. Or maybe she was stoned too.

I remember walking in the driveway with Danny, who was fumbling with a small package of white papers and a Baggie full of green leafy powder. He then lit a match, took a puff, and put this small, white, smoking twig in my mouth. It made me cough and gag when I followed his instructions to breathe in.

Was this a joke? Or did he want to share the life-sustaining magic with his baby brother?

I knew that the guillotine blade could drop from the medical board at any moment, yet, surreally, my day-to-day work life hadn't changed. Despite all of this chaos, I was still expected to show up every day, act chipper, enthusiastic, and empathic.

I had explained away Bruno and Rufus's visit by telling my colleagues that it related to the investigation of a drug-addicted patient. I didn't correct the general inference that this patient was someone other than me. My colleagues assumed it was the patient who had recently forged my signature on a computer-generated facsimile of my prescription pad. This came to light because the signature was that of a penmanship champion, in contrast to my trademark caveman scribbles.

On good days, being a primary care doctor isn't easy. It's not human nature to be that caring all day long. Mother Teresa would frazzle under a steady stream of needy patients, phone calls, insurance rejections, beeper pages, redundant paperwork, time pressure, and threats of litigation. She'd probably tune in, turn on, and drop out.

It was particularly difficult to concentrate with all the trouble I was dealing with. I neurotically ruminated about my predicament. Unless a patient was having a heart attack, I was more engrossed in my own problems. "Your knee hurts? Well, at least your whole life isn't screwed up. Depressed? About what? You gained five pounds? Big fucking deal. I'm facing financial ruin, divorce, and possibly, just possibly, prison time." It's fair to say that this was not an ideal therapeutic mind frame.

What was happening to me was enough to produce a panic attack in any Zen master. Even Lao Tzu would have become a neurasthenic who stuttered, smoked, and muttered to himself. Siddhartha would have drowned himself in my position. And they weren't sleeping on the sofa, trying to avoid a wife who zapped laser beams of hatred during every chance glimpse. Or withdrawing from narcotics.

Dressed in my white lab coat, examining patients, attending grand rounds, consulting with colleagues, ordering labs, all as if nothing had changed, I felt like an imposter, knowing it was soon going to end. I experienced a new awareness of the very transitoriness of my accomplishments in life.

Visually, my office, colleagues, staff, and patients all looked exactly the same, but I was seeing them through haunted eyes. For the two or three colleagues I was particularly close to, I was desperate to confess all, and to tell them what a fraud I was. I couldn't, because my drug seeking had involved them, as well as everyone else I knew.

Worst of all, I was desperately lonely. The only two people who knew what I was going through, excepting people connected in an official capacity, such as Bruno, Rufus, and Solomon, were H. and my twin brother, Martin. H. wasn't in a touchy-feely, communicative, lovey-dovey, nurturing frame of mind, so I didn't receive much emotional support. There was only so much my twin could do to help me. The only thing worse than going through something horrible is going through it alone.

H. started speaking to me, and about me, in a derogative manner. She introduced me as "the addict" or "my addict husband." She seemed to feel that it was a lack of spousal direction and control that had resulted in my becoming such a wayward husband. Clearly, I needed to be punished. When I made physical overtures to her, the answer wasn't "No" but "Are you joking?" What she really meant was "Never again." I sublimated this energy into all of the extra chores she was heaping on me.

Solomon told me to be especially careful with my narcotic prescriptions. He asked me to document carefully and to prescribe conservatively, so that the board couldn't claim I was still diverting them.

The morning after my court appearance, just as I was skulking up from the sofa to the bathroom, crawling up the creaky stairs and tiptoeing into the bedroom to avoid another drubbing by H., who was snoring softly, her red hair splayed across the pillow, my phone rang. I jumped up as if electrified, and muffled it with my hand. I heard an apologetic yet authoritative voice: "Hello, Dr. Grinspoon, this is Mattie from SHP calling. Today is a test day." I had until 4:00 p.m. I imagined Solomon's voice saying, "Don't flunk your drug test."

To ensure that my drug screens were legit, I was instructed to report to a Quest Diagnostics lab that had specialized procedures in place. This lab was on the second floor of a suburban office building in Brookline, Massachusetts. In the pale green waiting room, most of the other clients were blissed-out pregnant women being screened for gestational diabetes. How joyful they seemed by comparison. As they drank their red canisters labeled GLUCOSE, I guzzled as much water as possible to dilute the remaining molecules of the post–Bruno and Rufus Percocet.

The lab tech stepped out from behind the desk and bellowed "Number 1270," and I made my way forward. I was asked to show my ID, which does not have my name on it, just my number, like a prisoner number. I not only felt like a number, I *was* a number. My name never entered into the transaction. I was reminded of my elderly patients from my first practice out of residency, who were Holocaust survivors, with numbers tattooed on their arms, though I wouldn't presume to compare my plight to theirs.

I was informed that I wasn't allowed to wear a coat or any

baggy clothing that could conceal a Whizzinator. This was before the creators of the Whizzinator pleaded guilty to conspiracy to defraud the government by helping federal workers evade drug testing, and conspiracy to sell drug paraphernalia. That is a strange story about a weird invention. I was given a sealed plastic specimen cup and was monitored as I walked into the bathroom.

Once in the bathroom, I discovered that there was no running water, to prevent one of the clients from using water to dilute the sample. This made hand washing impossible. Gross. What pigs. There was blue dye in the toilet bowl to prevent us from using that water as well. My predecessors must have been desperate.

Once I finished and handed the cup to the nurse, they checked the temperature of the specimen to make sure it was at body temperature, not a smuggled-in sample, which would be cold. They would also check for soap and bleach, to make sure the sample wasn't spiked or damaged, and they check the concentration of the specimen to make sure I hadn't drunk excessive water beforehand.

Then came an elaborate ritual, sort of like signing your ketubah, which involves witnesses and signatures. They sealed the cup and put stickers on it, which I had to initial at each step to verify that I had watched the entire process and that it was done correctly. It is called "chain of custody" and it is meant to minimize the risk, given what's at stake, of a specimen getting labeled as someone else's. SHP then pretends the risk is zero, but it isn't. Just think of Annie Dookhan, who worked at the state lab in Massachusetts for years, deliberately falsifying samples.

This all took several hours, and I felt thoroughly degraded and humiliated, thinking "What kind of doctor has to do this?" I was externalizing my woes and blaming everyone else—the board, SHP, that stupid pharmacist that busted me—though deep down I knew that this was my fault and that I had bought and owned all of this guilt. If I didn't have a problem, none of this would be necessary, and my cheeks wouldn't be burning with shame as I walked out of the Quest laboratory.

I was late arriving at the office, which, in a primary care clinic, snowballs, because patients are grumpy that they've had to wait for you and then feel more justified in monopolizing your time, which gets you further behind. I barely finished the day in time to go to my first mandatory Narcotics Anonymous meeting.

One lasting result of Danny's successful use of cannabis is that the evil weed was invited into our household as a permanent guest of honor. My father, a Famous Psychiatrist, had recently published a book about marijuana, taking an increasingly pro-marijuana stance as he delved into the research and as he saw how it helped Danny. In 1972, this book was reviewed on the front page of the *New York Times Book Review*, which propelled my dad to hero status among potheads.

My father has always been an inspiration to me. He is an intellectual giant who came from poverty and managed to elevate himself into the highest echelons of academic life, both at Harvard Medical and beyond. He has exceptional integrity and has never been afraid to speak his mind or to go against the grain. He is largely responsible for the fact that cannabis is now legally available to millions of patients who desperately need it.

My dad had rushed to finish the book so that he could dedicate it to Danny before he died. The epigraph under the dedication reads, "Children are the greatest high of all."

Cannabis helped fill the vacuum in an atheistic family suffering such a large loss. We were in desperate need of something spiritual to latch onto. We had no church or temple, and no ideology beyond traditional liberal Jewish intellectual culture. What we stumbled upon in this time of distress was "Legalize it!" This became the cause célèbre that made Danny's death feel less meaningless.

My father believed that marijuana should be legalized for adults in the same way that alcohol is. The practical implication was that we remaining three boys were supposed to watch an endless parade of stoned adults traipsing through our house, having fun, spouting creative ideas, and acting silly, but not try it ourselves until adulthood.

Cannabis fit into and shaped the political culture of our family.

Wellesley, a suburb of Boston, was rich, right-wing, white, and WASP conservative, but in our house the spirit of the 1960s was still going strong. Our rooms were decorated with posters of the Grateful Dead and Hendrix. Danny's room was plastered with psychedelia from floor to ceiling. My parents left it like this for thirty years after he died, as a mausoleum.

My father's notoriety as a proponent of legalizing marijuana brought prominent elements of sixties counterculture directly into my childhood home.

When I was nine years old, a Famous Poet and his boyfriend were in our living room, discussing with my dad a campaign to free an imprisoned Russian dissident. I was supposed to be upstairs but, hearing the laughter and the merriment, I kept finding excuses to come down. By doing so, I was braving reprimand, but I knew this wouldn't be severe in front of company. It's hard to look like an enlightened leftist leader when you are clobbering your child.

Through a dense cloud of sticky smoke, the Famous Poet, throat dry, imperiously croaked, "Boy, get me some water." This was a far cry from "I saw the best minds of my generation destroyed by madness..." Even at age nine, I was flatly unimpressed.

On other occasions, my dad and a Famous Astronomer would be passing around the hookah. They discussed complex philosophical issues, such as why the workingman still clings to religious beliefs when science fully explains the universe. As they smoked and talked, and talked and smoked, the Famous Astronomer ate billions and billions of appetizers.

When I was nine, these adults seemed godlike in their knowledge and in their confidence. As I listened to these genuinely brilliant cannabis-fueled conversations, it seemed as if Very Important Things were happening in our living room. It encouraged me to read everything I could get my hands on, and to try my hardest in school, so I could also be one of the intellectual giants of the world.

My first Narcotics Anonymous meeting was held in the basement/dungeon of the Shattuck, a run-down hospital of last resort for prisoners, the criminally insane, and the desperately poor. The meeting took place in a dicey area of working-class, ethnically mixed Jamaica Plain, about a mile from where I first met H. seven years earlier. My addiction counselor, Ben, his voice raspy from hypocritically chain-smoking cigarettes, tried to warn me away from this particular meeting: "It's too rough and it's a drug bazaar." Gee, that sounds terrible. Where do I sign up?

When I arrived, I felt nervous and out of place, as there were dozens of recovering addicts, mostly Hispanic and African American, including several different groups of heavily tattooed gang members who eyed me warily. I should have dressed down after work. Somehow my tie and shirt clashed with their tattoos. Participants were asked to leave their weapons outside. Luckily, I had left my rocket launcher at home.

Incarcerated patients under guard added to what I initially perceived as an ambience of thuggery and sociopathy. Until the week before, I was an elite physician who would have had nothing to do with these people, except if I were volunteering in a clinic for homeless addicts.

The meeting, once the chaos was tamed enough to allow it to begin, was supportive and cooperative, with lots of applause, hugs, and boisterous yells of encouragement. It presented an overwhelming mélange of contrasting stereotypes. I was feeling utterly adrift until I was elbowed and a friendly, familiar voice whispered to me, "Hey, Doc, you on the juice too?" It was Frank, my cheerful neighborhood barber, who was also a patient of mine. He pulled up a chair for me. Feeling vastly more comfortable, I settled in for the ride.

When it was time for me to introduce myself, with dozens of pairs of expectant and skeptical eyes gazing at me, it was impossible for me to more than mumble the simple, required mantra: "My name is Peter, and I'm an addict."

I hadn't even begun to understand or embrace my new identity. These meetings seemed to have nothing to do with me. They were concerned with drug addicts and street people. I assumed the role of the lofty anthropologist studying a culture of criminality and vice, and tried to radiate a kindly but patronizing smile.

The meeting quickly became boring, with too much God talk from desperate people who had seen the light in prison. They all seemed brainwashed. After all I had been through that week, I was *not* in the mood for this. I'd rather be stuck in an elevator listening to Muzak than talking about God. I'd rather be smashing rocks in Siberia.

Indignant that I had to suffer through this misplaced religiosity, I next tried an AA meeting in a church in blue-collar West Roxbury, thinking I'd get back to the proletarian roots of my immigrant forebears. Despite five years of dealing with angry, bomb-throwing communists while working at Greenpeace, I was about as proletarian as Imelda Marcos.

To my disappointment, I didn't relate at all to these earnest, religious, old-school, AA recovering alcoholics. Their language wasn't crisp, and they repeated slogans over and over again. Someone would say, "Let go and let God," and everyone would nod enthusiastically or start cheering. Their thoughts were fuzzy. They all seemed to be heartened and sustained by something I couldn't perceive, as if they were all breathing nitrous and I was breathing regular old oxygen.

I was going to be required to attend these meetings for years, and I had to choose between gang/druggie God talk and fuzzy alcoholic God talk. Help! Maybe I should just surrender myself to the medical board.

Some systems require proof of attendance at support group meetings. Drunk drivers on probation, for example, have to ask the meeting director to sign a slip of paper after the meeting is over. SHP uses the honor system, and I ended up going to Starbucks instead of the meetings, and reading novels. H. had to allow me to leave the house, because the meetings were required. I'd come home at just the time I would return from a meeting. I reasoned that reading *David Copperfield* was more germane to my spiritual recovery than the Christian god was.

Regardless of my aesthetic critique of these meetings and their content, there was no way for me to avoid being railroaded into the next phase of my evaluation. With a heavy heart, I started packing for my trip to the Talbott Recovery Center in Atlanta.

I was gearing up for what I believed would essentially be a five-day-long Alcoholics Anonymous meeting. I had only a thin shield of atheism, the tattered remains of my self-esteem, and an abundance of skepticism to hide behind.

Like most teens, we had access to our parents' liquor closet, but the first time I tried alcohol, at age twelve, I got sick and learned my lesson. We drank my dad's scotch, which felt good at first, and then turned on me. Swimming in nausea, I crawled into my parents' bedroom, a very bad choice, and barfed all over their wall and rug. Ever charitable and trusting, my mom said, "Poor Peter has food poisoning." The smell of scotch still makes me sick, and alcohol is one drug I've never had trouble turning down.

More enticing was our access to my dad's reefer supply. He kept small stuffed plastic bags barely hidden, in the back of a drawer or behind a speaker. It didn't occur to him that teenagers are expert snoops and that we might pilfer it.

My first deliberate marijuana experience was at age twelve, on the same Cape Cod beach where we spread Danny's ashes. I briefly wondered what Danny would have thought. Would he have chuckled, "The twins are smoking reefer," or would he have been prescient enough, having grown in the five years since his death, to see what all this was going to lead to?

Our marijuana use was meticulously planned, good practice for direct actions at Greenpeace ten years later. The weed was secreted out of our dad's supply gradually, so he wouldn't notice. An elementary wooden pipe was bought several weeks earlier in Provincetown, at one of the many head shops still legally open back then. This pipe was rectangular, with a small square storage compartment built into the stem, which slid open and shut. The buds were in there, patiently waiting, biding their time.

We picked a day when my parents were off sailing and couldn't possibly return to the beach for at least several hours.

Martin, our friend Will, and I huddled together in the dunes, where we had grown up, innocent kids building sand castles and body surfing, fending off the "sand and water treatment," a friendly torture where an older, stronger cousin or sibling dunks you in the water and then rolls you in the sand, pinning you down while the sun bakes the sand onto your skin. The other cousins would all stand up and cheer while this was happening, as if we were in a Roman coliseum. It would itch and burn for days.

Flattened down against the wind and the drizzle, I felt an intoxicating blend of nervousness and anticipation. We didn't know how to inhale or even how to light the pipe. We also didn't know that the first time you smoke, nothing happens. We spent the next several hours asking ourselves if we were high. This new ritual felt cool and important, a rite of passage for us to enter the world of adults. Sort of like an atheist stoner's version of a bar mitzvah.

With the wind and the drizzle, we had trouble lighting the pipe. Forgetting to blow out the match, I set fire to my shirt, which was lying on the beach. I couldn't believe that my damp shirt caught fire so easily, when we were having no luck with this stubborn pipe. The incineration of my shirt was a foreshadowing of what stronger drugs would later do to my life.

It was chilly in the rain, so I wore this shirt home, deliberately nonchalant about the two-inch circular burn mark on the back, hoping that no one would notice until I had time to change. I should have written off the shirt as a total loss and made it disappear, because my story about someone walking into me while smoking a cigarette wasn't quite plausible to my parents, who were starting to intuit that we were sneaks, up to no good. My story was non-falsifiable, so they let it drop, but even my credulous mother was, for the first time, skeptical of me, and greeted me with something uncharacteristically sarcastic.

As meticulously described in *The Tennis Partner* by Abraham Verghese, the Talbott Center is an inpatient rehab facility that specializes in treating health care professionals. SHP sent me for a more in-depth evaluation of whether I needed the full ninety-day rehab package with bells and whistles.

The problem at this point was that I was still blaming everyone and everything else for what I was going through: Work was so stressful, H. was such an unforgiving bitch, and it was exhausting being a parent to two small children. Never did it dawn on me to take even some of the responsibility for what was happening. This was my frame of mind as I flew down to Talbott in Atlanta to fulfill the week-long inpatient part of my SHP contract.

From the second I landed, I was in get-out-of-rehab mode. I became a mechanized propaganda machine, reciting whatever words were necessary to avoid being committed, and I mean committed, to ninety days of this. How could I put my life on hold for ninety days? This was unspeakable. I wanted to keep working and try to reconcile with H., not sit in Atlanta, roasting in the heat with these loser fuckups while my life further unraveled at home. I still thought that the addiction was under my control, and that it was only due to a careless misstep and bad luck that I got caught.

I spouted about my commitment to recovery to the friendly addicts who picked me up at the airport, to the psychiatrist who evaluated me, to the addiction counselors who interviewed me, to anyone who would listen. "I understand what I did wrong, that I'm addicted, that I need to change my behavior and my coping strategies. Really, I do. I am powerless over this and I will ask my higher power to help me." The psychiatrist, who looked young enough to still be in medical school, didn't buy my act at all. "You are in denial, you need help, and you need it for a long time." She wanted to throw away the key. Another unforgiving bitch.

My roommate, Demitri, was a sociopath internist who was battling federal methamphetamine charges. His protestations of innocence clanged hollow. I hoped I didn't sound that phony. The other patients struck me as hopeless cases as well. They were all cynically doing their time to mollify their medical and nursing boards. They spent every moment of free time vacantly staring at the television instead of exploring their recovery, exercising, meditating, reading, or talking. It reminded me of the medicated zombies in the psych ward at medical school. I would wither and die if I had to be here for ninety days.

Sometimes hard work is rewarded. Despite a harsh minority

opinion from the psychiatrist, the Talbott assessment was that I "deserve a chance to pursue recovery as an outpatient." Dodged that bullet, or so I thought. I almost danced for joy. Can't touch this.

Despite my status at home as the deep-shit, doghouse dad, I savored seeing and feeling my kids rush into my arms in an ecstatic welcome. For now, at least, I knew that I wouldn't be separated from them. I could take comfort in the knowledge that our nightly rituals of drenching bubble baths and reading from Disney picture books would continue. This is one thing that the addiction hadn't taken away from me.

I flew home just in time to depart for a cruise with H.'s family in the Caribbean. I asked Solomon if I needed permission to leave the country, and he said, "No, that's fine, just don't come back and flunk a drug test."

This vacation, with H.'s parents, sister, her fiancé, and Annie and Milo, on a confined cruise ship in the Caribbean, couldn't possibly have been more poorly timed. It was as if God were punishing me for being an unbeliever. I'd rather be burned at the stake by the pagan hordes than imprisoned on a boat with H. just after my prescription violation. I would have walked the plank if there had been one.

There was no getting out of this, because her parents had already paid for it and because H. didn't want to let her parents know that anything was wrong with the doctor she had proudly harpooned seven years earlier.

Packing for trips was the most stressful aspect of my marriage with H. Even without two small children, it was almost impossible to get out the door, because she would insist on repacking multiple times and on cleaning up the house to spotlessness before we left. Annie and Milo packed enough stuffed animals to populate Antarctica, and cried piteously when we limited them to two apiece.

Like an endangered polar bear flushed from his shrinking Arctic habitat, I was denied the refuge of the living room sofa and was stuck in a small cabin with H. This made the scenario painted by Sartre in *No Exit* look like *Barney & Friends* in comparison. Hell is other people.

During the cruise, H. mostly yelled at me in private, was affectionate in public, and gave me detailed childcare instructions before she went off to relax. During these lectures, I gazed out the small oval porthole, which was our only window. I pondered if, by starving myself for the rest of the voyage, I could stuff myself through this window and drown.

The whole cruise ship was more like a floating marital doghouse, leaving in its wake a trail of floating dog hair, chew toys, and splintered bits of my soul. From the second I set foot on ship, I started to wish that I had been locked up in Talbott instead. Maybe the psychiatrist at Talbott was a prescient genius like Dr. Stern. I wanted to call her back and say, "You're right, I'm on drugs, lock me up. Can you please send a helicopter right away?"

My mental state was in stark contrast to that of the other passengers, who ate, drank colorful cocktails, danced, gambled, laughed, and snuggled up next to their loving and supportive partners. I felt about as festive as the bleak and hopeless protagonist in Dostoyevsky's *Notes from the Underground*.

I remember swimming with giant stingrays in shallow, sandy water, walking up a large tropical waterfall with a stone staircase carved into the center, and sea kayaking with H. Not one of these memories is stored in a part of my brain with neural connections to pleasant or relaxing associations. H. acted out her anger at me by loudly criticizing my rowing and navigation skills while we were kayaking. "You just don't know how to paddle, do you? More to the left. Harder. No, I said to the right." (Subtext: you druggie asshole.)

We had just come from Jamaica, where in the space of an hour, at least a dozen people approached us with "Some reefer, mon?" Desperate as I was to float away in great clouds of soothing smoke, I didn't think this was a good idea for a variety of reasons, including death by wife, flunking my SHP tests, and risking arrest by an undercover cop posing as a drug dealer. Even Solomon wouldn't be able to bring me home in one piece.

We were visiting a colorful outdoor market and shopping area on one of the Caribbean islands. I couldn't take H.'s angry criticisms anymore, and I was feeling overwhelmingly dejected. I decided to do some island exploration on my own.

"H., I'm going to go back to that hat store and try to find a more comfortable hat. I'll meet you over at that fountain in fifteen minutes."

"Don't take more than ten minutes and don't spend more than fifteen dollars. Don't go anywhere else."

Next to the hat store was a pharmacy, which I had noticed within seconds of our arriving, because this is the kind of thing that lights up the receptors in my brain. I knew from previous travels in the third world that controlled medications/drugs are often sold without prescriptions. To my disappointment, in this particular country, because of the long, bullying arm of the DEA, nothing much was available.

The best I could do was about eight pills of Suboxone, which is a mild narcotic used for detoxing people off heroin. I bought them for $120 and swallowed them on the spot so they wouldn't show up if H. decided to strip-search me. At that point, that was the only stripping we were doing together. So far from home, in a different world, I put it out of my mind that, back in Boston in a few days, SHP would be calling me for a drug screen.

The vacation was over in a flash, and soon we were riding in a cab, back to our home in Hyde Park. H. and I were sitting in an uncomfortable silence, and we each had a child snoozing on our laps. Neither of us tried to make conversation. The soft snoring of our children filled me with hope that possibly, just possibly, things were going to be OK. Dark foreboding would have been more appropriate and accurate.

As we grew up, our idolatry of our older brother, David, knew no bounds. He exerted a magnetic, if not entirely wholesome, influence on us as we entered the early teen years. He attended Brown University, and he sported a Jewfro that extended out at least eight inches from his skull. The combined diameter of his hair and head was about two feet.

David was a creative and inclusive older brother, happy to still have some siblings left in his life. As we rode Amtrak by ourselves from Boston to Providence to visit him on weekends, we left the bullying and the unpopularity that we faced in junior high school behind. With an increasing sense of excitement, we ascended the hill from which Brown overlooked the polluted squalor of Providence.

Did my parents believe we were going to be supervised when we visited David? By whom? Surely they didn't trust David to do this. Did they envision us being exposed to good influences, such as watching David and his friends read and learn in the halls of this august Ivy League institution?

At Brown, David lived in Carberry, the hippiest of hippie dorms, with group meals, coed showers, long hair and beards, free love, and unlimited drugs. No modesty. Wild dancing. Blaring Hendrix. Inedible vegetable mush for dinner. People openly snorting cocaine, smoking joints, inhaling nitrous, and saying things like, "I'm tripping so hard; do you think if I smoke some pot it will help me come down?" I stored all of these insights on my internal hard drive for later reflection and emulation.

In seventh grade, I remember it being impossible to concentrate on an English test with the few brain cells that had survived the previous night's Grateful Dead concert, our first.

We had taken the early morning train back from visiting David at Brown. The Grateful Dead concert, absorbed through twelve-year-old sensory apparatus, was earth-shattering. We sat in the eighteenth row, center stage. Aptly, it started with the song "Promised Land." We passed the dutchie but didn't inhale.

We stayed up most of the night and ate a midnight dinner at the clamorous dining room of my brother's off-campus hippie dorm house, more of the textureless vegetable mush. We slept on the floor.

Most of my brother's friends were on acid and were staring out into space. Someone dared my brother to dance around the room with underwear on his head, which was readily taken off and handed to him by one of the sultry, hallucinating hippie chicks. This dance was a masterpiece of pure silliness. We boarded an early morning Amtrak train in order to make it back to junior high school on time.

The experience of this concert, the drugs, and our brother's friends, who treated us like entertaining pets, not junior high school rejects, suggested to us a meaning and purpose beyond the day-to-day, a purposefulness that was wholly lacking in the dull hallways of our school, where kids bullied and boasted about nothing.

The other kids at Wellesley Junior High School, who were taking this same English test alongside us, went to Little League practice the night before, ate in a civilized manner at well-set tables with their families, and then enjoyed a good night's sleep. In a bed. With pajamas. No sultry, hallucinating hippie chicks surrendering their underwear. Is it any wonder that we didn't fit in? At least I aced the English test.

By age fourteen, unsupervised at Carberry, we would smoke and smoke until we were only nominally more substantial than the rest of the atmosphere. As we wandered around as if in a dream, glassy-eyed, nonverbal, and starving, the other students at Carberry interacted with us in the same way people treat a cute new puppy. When stoned at age fourteen, merely walking down the block to get pizza in a strange city is an all-encompassing sensory adventure. Eating the plainest of food was a transcendent experience.

From our early teenage vantage point, this world was impossibly fun and magical, especially compared with the mindlessness and conformity of our concurrent junior high experience. Away from the bullying and the rigid dress, language, and behavior expectations of our middle school, we were able to forge our own identities.

Because of the messages we perceived, growing up in our particular childhood home, we believed that smoking marijuana was entirely harmless. By toking, we were carrying on the fight of the sixties against imperialism, racism, sexism, and fascism. We were finally participating in the intellectual elite, arm in arm with the Famous Poets, Astronomers, and Psychiatrists of this world.

Driving home from work on the second week back from the Caribbean, having survived a twelve-hour marathon of patient visits, e-mails, calls, pages, and lab results, interrupted by a drug test, all while feeling like my time on Earth as a doctor was running out, my cell rang with a private number. "You are a *major-league* fuckup. I told you not to flunk a drug test."

It was my ever-sensitive attorney Solomon, telling me that I was utterly screwed with the medical board. Fear and panic notwithstanding, it hurt my feelings that he called me a fuckup. Imagine paying $400 an hour for someone to call you a fuckup. Solomon then instructed me to send him an even bigger retainer and said, most insultingly of all, "You're becoming my annuity."

SHP had just informed Solomon that my urine test had turned up with Valium in it. I couldn't believe it. There must be some mistake. How unfair. This is not even remotely possible. Those screwups said they were careful not to switch the specimens. There needs to be a retest immediately.

I prepared to launch these defenses, though there wasn't a snowball's chance in hell that even Solomon, whom I pay, and who specializes in this field, would buy it. According to Solomon, "Even if you were innocent, which you clearly aren't, an addict denying drug use holds no water."

I gave up the fight because I knew that I had been illicitly taking Valium from a large supply I had stored up over the previous few months, having siphoned them from a patient. I was taking Valium in addition to Klonapin, which my psychiatrist had been prescribing for sleep. I rationalized that if Klonapin was OK, then so was Valium. I'm a doctor who knows what he's doing. There's extra stress in my life. What merciless pricks would begrudge me this? Whose business was it?

At the hospitals where I worked, the drug screens were less sensitive and specific than the SHP drug screens. According to the tests I was used to, my legitimate Klonapin use should have covered up the illicit Valium, because the two chemicals are so similar. In our lab, they would be indistinguishable.

I had vastly underestimated the SHP system, which is specifically designed for wily doctors who go to great lengths, using the full force of their scientific expertise, to cheat these tests. The SHP drug screen goes several steps further and is able to discern between these two similar drugs because they produce different breakdown products. I had no defense.

I didn't at that point understand how costly this failed test would prove for my future, besides involving a lot more money for Solomon, though I was filled with enough foreboding by this news that I had to pull my cluttered Subaru off the road in order to take some deep breaths.

With trembling fingers, I dialed my addiction counselor, Ben. He picked up on the first ring, as if he were waiting by the phone. "Peter, we knew this might happen. It's part of addiction. Your denial is tripping you up. You aren't honest. Take responsibility for this like an adult. Go to rehab." I thought, "Fuck you very much" and hung up the phone.

This positive test started a dreamlike sequence of rapidly escalating events, a chain reaction of ever more painful and long-lasting consequences.

In the wake of the positive test, Solomon walked me through the steps of surrendering my medical license, resigning from my job, and trying to head off criminal charges that were now even more serious because I no longer had recourse to the "I've learned from my mistakes" defense. He informed me that I might have to go away to rehab for three months to show the medical board and the courts how serious I was about recovery. He told me to report to the office of the medical board at 8:00 the next morning. (Again with the 8:00 a.m. mandatory reporting!)

The medical board's office was located in the basement of a row house in a run-down area squeezed between two very different Boston neighborhoods, the gay and festive South End and the destitute minority neighborhood of Roxbury. It is situated adjacent to the Boston Medical Center campus, where I had graduated from medical school eight years earlier, at the top of my class, a rising star.

I associated this part of Boston with sleepless nights in the hospital, late-night gorging in Chinatown with classmates, marathon study sessions, and ecstatic celebration after matching at a top residency program in primary care. Mostly, I associated it with my idealism as a medical student, planning a lifelong career of selflessly caring for people and of ongoing scholarship.

It was with a very different feeling that I walked with Solomon down the steps into the fluorescent brightness of these basement offices. Captured by the Romans, I was being led in a chain and collar to the coliseum. These lights illuminated the inside of my brain, all the way to the back of my skull.

The staff was friendly and polite: "Oh, hi, Dr. Grinspoon, we'll be with you in a moment," as if I were waiting for a meeting with my financial adviser or a travel agent, though underneath, I sensed a hint of censoriousness.

Waiting in the lobby, I bumped into one of my heroes from medical school, Juan, who, as chief resident, had been one of my instructors and mentors. He was a dynamic and caring doctor, involved with social programs to help impoverished patients. He was at the board helping two new residents with a minor snag in their paperwork.

Unable to render myself invisible, I walked over to Juan and exchanged pleasantries, but was evasive when he asked what I was doing there. How could I explain this? I managed a weak smile and moved on, reeling from how far I had come down in the world.

My meeting with the board's attorney was brief, because my disposition had been negotiated in advance by Solomon. In a somber ceremony, I signed a "voluntary agreement not to practice medicine," which, though not technically a suspension, was similar in that my license was active. I now needed a ruling by the medical board to practice medicine again. It gave them reassurance that I wouldn't put any patients at risk.

Signing this document, I felt like crying, the tears washing away all my hard work and all of my hopes for the future. But I was determined not to blubber in front of these attorneys, because I needed to maintain a shred of my dignity. I was a doctor now only in name. Professionally gelded. Knocked off my godlike perch.

I envisioned myself padding around the house, still in pajamas midday, unshaven, unkempt, perhaps smoking cigarettes again, picking the kids up from preschool and packing their lunches. Waiting for contractors. Picking up the dry cleaning. Receiving daily "honey do" lists from H. Criticized nightly for not completing them. The highlight of my day would be my pilgrimage to leave a urine sample for SHP.

Stay-at-home dad/nanny/handyman/housecleaner/personal assistant to a mercurial wife was a steep fall from successful internist and faculty member at Preparation H (aka Harvard). How would I explain all of this to friends, relatives, colleagues, and acquaintances? Just thinking about it caused my cheeks to flame.

This arrangement with the board spared me the humiliation and publicity of being suspended, though the board did place a press release on their website detailing my infractions and the disciplinary action rendered. This publicity had widespread implications later on, including tarnishing my reputation with both my colleagues and my patients and making it more difficult, much later, to find employment.

The fact that we always had abundant weed, obtained from my brother David's friends or from my dad's reefer closet, gained us entrance into the upper echelons of high school druggie culture. We experimented with magic mushrooms as well.

Once we tried to buy pot on the Boston Common. We approached two African American teenagers, who told us that they would sell us some reefer if we gave them twenty dollars each. "We'll be back with your stash in a few minutes." As they continued walking across the common, with no intention of coming back, receding into the distance, we realized that we were idiots who weren't as sophisticated as we would have liked to believe.

Why weren't we supervised? It's amazing what you can get away with if you have top grades. This fact alone kept our other activities off the parental radar.

Though my parents didn't appear to be entirely abstemious either. The night before the SAT, Martin had to put a towel under the door of my parents' bedroom, because my parents, along with the Famous Astronomer and his wife, were hunkered in their bedroom, behind a locked door, with marijuana smoke billowing out. We wished to avoid getting a contact high the night before our big exam.

As high school went on, with increasingly popular and well-attended pot parties, a deafening if somewhat atonal rock band, academic success, and a hot Australian girlfriend for me, we came to feel, with the narcissism of teenagers, that we were the leaders of a small countercultural revolution in our high school. The Sandinistas had nothing on us. We had succeeded, at least for ourselves, in linking our home culture with the outside world.

In my own internal crucible, I blended influences and impressions, such as the dizzying discussions I overheard with the Famous Astronomer, the peak experiences I was having on pot and shrooms, the book *Zen and the Art of Motorcycle Maintenance*, and the meaningless brevity of Danny's life. I found that I had my own thoughts on how to live my life: Accumulate as many intense experiences as possible, because tomorrow it may all be gone. I called this philosophy "Danny and the Art," as metaphor for all that I suspected was out there for me to discover, to observe, and, eventually, to form.

When I was accepted to Swarthmore College, a superintense, alternative, leftist liberal arts college in Pennsylvania, I felt that the Door Had Opened. But as I was transitioning to this next phase, I started to get glimpses of some of the casualties that went along with our "revolution." Most ominous was what happened to Will, our initial pot pal.

One evening, when Martin and I, along with Martin's girlfriend, were visiting Will at his dorm, I decided to try the acid (LSD) he offered us. I found this to be a deeply pleasurable experience: The world exploding into an unimaginable kaleidoscope of colors, regardless of whether my eyes were open or closed. An American flag flapping on the wall of his room, as if in a steady breeze, though the windows were closed in the dead of winter.

Driving back to our parents' house in Wellesley, Martin, the designated driver, stone-cold sober, managed to miss a turn and drive in the wrong direction on Commonwealth Avenue for a brief stretch. I would have done a better job driving on acid.

Once we returned to my parents' house, Will disappeared for a while, then was seen walking up the stairs, dressed in his birthday suit, covered only by Martin's girlfriend's unbuttoned overcoat. He suddenly lurched toward her and tried to throw her down the stairs. After this, he locked himself in my bedroom and started smashing things. Large things. Holy shit.

After a desperate consultation with Martin, it was decided that I would be the one to seek help, despite the fact that I was still tripping, because I was the more fearless and persuasive. I went into my parents' room, woke them up at 2:00 a.m., and said, "Um, er...excuse me. We can discuss this in more detail later, but Will says that he took some LSD and now he's lost his mind and is locked in my bedroom smashing things." This statement was punctuated by a large crash, as Will tipped over a dresser.

My dad came over to the locked door of my room. He used his deep, commanding parental/psychiatric/Harvard command voice that *no one* ignores. "Will, this is Dr. Lester Grinspoon. Unlock the door *right now*." This had no effect whatsoever on Will.

Out of options, and concerned for Will's safety, my parents called the police, who put Will in a straitjacket and brought him to Newton-Wellesley Hospital. While they were subduing him, I was flushing the rest of the acid down the toilet. When the police questioned me, I played dumb and managed to give a coherent cover story, even though the white part of one officer's eyes was bluish purple and his face was slightly molten. "He came over tonight and seemed to be on some kind of drug."

The drive over to the hospital was surreal, only partially because of the lingering effects of the LSD. My father was feeling frustrated and misunderstood, as well as furious. He said, "If you had only read my book on psychedelic drugs, you would know

that this kind of thing can happen." Through ziggy lines of dancing oxygen molecules, I shot back: "What do you expect us to do?
All we hear about at home is how interesting this stuff is. I did
read your book. It's all about how cool these drugs are, and how
'altered states' are better."

The deliberately guilt-inducing "I'm a victim of the messages
I've received from you" defense was partially successful, and our
punishment for this episode was modest at best.

After a few hours at Newton-Wellesley Hospital, Will, with
the help of sedatives and restraints, was feeling somewhat less
violent. We were met there by his dad, a neurologist, and his new
stepmom, an image-conscious social climber who gave us a with-
eringly reproachful glare, as if to warn us off from further inter-
fering with her future aspirations for this new stepson.

I was extremely shaken up by Will's acid-induced freak-out.
Up until this point, it had only been fun and games. There
weren't any consequences to our drug use, except that we were
becoming popular in high school. In a flash, we were dealing
with some near-deadly consequences. My best friend was entirely
transformed, by this small tab of paper that we had put under our
tongues several hours earlier, from a happy and carefree jokester
into a psychotic fiend who needed to be restrained and sedated in
a hospital. If only I had paid attention to this.

After my slaughter at the hands of the medical board, we walked
back up the steps to Solomon's Lexus convertible, of which I
had already paid for at least the steering wheel and several of the
tires. Solomon said, "You realize, don't you, that you need to go
to rehab, starting as soon as possible, for at least three months, to
have any chance of reversing this? This is nonnegotiable."

I had been resisting the idea of rehab with every molecule of
my body. I would rather spend ninety days in a Siberian labor
camp, choking down black bread, starving, freezing, abused by
guards, patching together worn-out clothing to ward off frost-
bite. Ninety days in the life of Peter Grinspoon.

Over the last six months, Ben and my psychiatrist had been

frequently threatening to report me to the medical board as an impaired physician. That might have spared me Hurricane Rufus, if only I hadn't ignored their warnings. They had also been suggesting an inpatient rehab stint.

Rehab was also being insisted upon by Dr. T., a substance abuse guru in my hospital, with whom I had a desperate encounter several months earlier. I had sought out Dr. T. a few days after my patient Paul had left a bottle of almost five hundred eighty-milligram oxycodone tablets in my office.

Paul had returned the pills to me in protest because, he insisted, only the brand-name Oxycontin, not the generic oxycodone, alleviated his back pain. These two formulations are virtually identical in chemical composition, but Oxycontin has a vastly higher street value. Two bucks a milligram translates into tens of thousands of dollars per prescription. My suspicions were compounded by having bumped into a pain-free and spry Paul the previous summer.

Paul has blond hair, is skinny, and is meticulously polite. In my office, he invariably limped, clutched his back, and groaned loudly in agony due to his "back pain." Paul was on a gigantic dose of Oxycontin, higher than any patient I've had to this day, which I continued from his previous doctor. At that point in my career, I didn't look at these cases nearly as critically as I do now, possibly because back then I was abusing the same pills.

That summer, I was visiting Cape Cod with H. As we were walking hand in hand on an obscure gravel pathway, known from my childhood, down to the area where my brother Danny's ashes were scattered, I saw, of all people, Paul walking toward us. He was effortlessly carrying an obviously heavy box, walking without a limp, healthy, hearty, and carefree. He had been limping and groaning in my office the week before.

When he noticed me, he didn't bother with the limp or the groans. Instead, he offered a friendly smile and handshake. "Hey, Doc, how are you? Imagine bumping into you here." He cheerfully invited us to go sailing with him on his thirty-footer.

How could someone with constant, excruciating back pain, requiring hundreds of milligrams of Oxycontin, sail a large boat?

Hauling rope, lifting the anchor, pulling the rudder, loading supplies. I doubted his diminutive-looking wife could do all that, unless she was a Romanian weightlifter on steroids.

In retrospect, at two-dollars-per-milligram street value, the Oxycontin is possibly what paid for the yacht in the first place. He might have been unsatisfied with the generic prescription because he still had payments to make. In essence, he was saying, "You inconsiderate doctor, how do you expect me to maintain my yacht and summerhouse with only *generic* medication to pawn?"

Having been left this bounty of rejected pills in my office, I brought them home, and after H. finally fell asleep, I took five of them. I can't remember what happened next. When I woke up, I was more disoriented than I'd ever been, and it took me a while to piece together what I had swallowed the night before. I knew that I could have turned permanently blue in my sleep, only to be found in the morning by H., who wouldn't know which to do first, yell at me or cry. The *Boston Globe* headline: HARVARD DOCTOR OVERDOSES IN BED. PRONOUNCED DEAD BEFORE WIFE HAD CHANCE TO KILL HIM.

When I was coherent enough to do some belated calculations, I realized that I had taken the equivalent of eighty Percocet tablets. (Each eighty-milligram oxycodone tablet was equivalent to sixteen five-milligram Percocets.) On a bad day, at the height of my addiction, I might take ten or possibly fifteen Percocets, but not eighty. Never eighty.

These megapills were just too strong. I knew that I wouldn't be able to stop taking them and that I would be dead long before the remaining pills were gone. Acting according to some primitive survival instinct, I brought them to Dr. T. to dispose of. This was a big step, because it was admitting, for the first time, that I didn't have this situation entirely under control.

Dr. T. is a tall, slightly portly man in his early sixties, with graying hair and a pleasant, humble demeanor. He has a well-earned reputation for being empathic, judicious, and nonjudgmental, though tough as nails when need be. He is a prominent expert on substance abuse and was well aware of my case because Ben had consulted with him, believing that I was a meltdown waiting to happen.

To me, he had extra credibility, because he survived and overcame an addiction himself, which had landed him in all kinds of deep shit as a young man.

Dr. T. was welcoming and cordial as I entered his office, though I could tell he had his bullshit detectors turned up to eleven. "Dr. T., I need your help. You know from Ben that I'm struggling with addiction. If you don't get rid of these pills, they're going to be the end of me." I dramatically flourished the full bottle of large pills. "I'll be one of those tragic cases people read about in the newspaper. These people will shake their heads and say 'what a waste.' My wife will say 'I told you so.' It will break my parents' hearts. Can you help me?"

"Peter, I'm glad you came in and, yes, I can help you."

He took the bottle from me and, as he was flushing the pills down the toilet in his private office, he claimed, to make me feel better, "I've flushed bigger bottles than this." I doubted this, given that the bottle contained enough opiates to sedate the entire hospital. Once these were flushed, there were going to be some very stoned fish in Boston Harbor.

There were so many large pills, I was worried about clogging the toilet and causing an Oxycontin flood in the hospital, dripping opiate euphoria and sewage onto the floor below.

As a fee for his service, I had to listen to a long, detailed explanation of how I needed to take an immediate leave of absence and go to rehab. Short of this, he predicted I would end up stripped of my medical license and possibly behind bars, as he once had been, if I survived at all.

He prescribed me Suboxone, which is the new methadone for getting people off opiates. He said that he would try the Suboxone once, on the remote possibility that I could turn it around without rehab. A few months later, hooked again, I came crawling back for more and he turned me away, which couldn't have been easy for him.

My response to these earlier suggestions that I go to rehab was straightforward: absolutely not. The very idea seemed like hysteria, overkill. The humiliation would be unbearable. At the time, I didn't think I could leave my practice, my marriage, or my kids for even a few days. H. couldn't manage the house, and the kids would forget who I was. Three months was a lifetime to them.

I had a taste of rehab at Talbott, and there was a snowball's chance in hell that I'd willingly go through it again, with that patronizing bitch psychiatrist and all the arbitrary rules and the hopeless, sociopathic people I had to deal with.

My ongoing fantasy of rehab was of some medieval place, cut off from modern society, where my personality would be beaten out of me, to be supplanted by a robotic allegiance to some faith-based recovery program. (As it turns out, this fantasy was dead-on accurate.) Nothing in my Talbott experience did anything to improve this impression. I was convinced that rehab was for rich fuckup lushes with too much time on their hands, and trust-fund hippies who had done too much acid. I hadn't done acid for years, and I wasn't living off a trust fund. You've got the wrong guy!

I pleaded my case with Ben, thinking he could explain to Solomon, and to the medical board, that I was such an exemplar of serious recovery in our therapy sessions that I didn't even need rehab, that rehab would be redundant with my monk-like commitment to abstinence. I was practically begging. Practically? I was groveling.

Through the haze of his chain-smoking and my frazzled neurons, I pleaded my case. The verdict: "Peter, you are full of shit. You have more denial than anyone I've ever treated. You are acting like a teenager, but you aren't a teenager. You are in your thirties, with a wife and kids. You have to grow up. Patients depend on you. You have to pull it together, and stop digging yourself into a deeper hole. Rehab is exactly what you need, for as long as possible. They should throw away the key. And if you raise a fuss, I'm going to stick a boot up your ass."

In other words, he agreed with Solomon. At this juncture, the only path to follow to beat the rap, for the courts to back off, to have a chance of avoiding a criminal record, to eventually retrieve my medical license, to regain all that I had lost, was to go to rehab.

I would depart for rehab at Tannenberg Rehab in North Carolina in two weeks' time.

Within weeks of my arrival at Swarthmore College, I joined most of the student body in protesting a 1984 campaign visit by Ronald Reagan to Philadelphia. Downtown Philly was packed, and the crowd was not particularly sympathetic to the Walter Mondale placards we were brandishing. One of my fellow students, an immature provocateur, was standing right next to me when he yelled, "Let's set that large flag on fire!" and we were chased down the block by an angry mob, who yelled "communist" and "traitor."

The crowd was almost exclusively blue-collar Caucasians, a segment of society that was becoming steadily less prosperous under Reagan. They were still waiting for the fruits of life to trickle down to them, like Linus waiting for the Great Pumpkin to appear.

During his first term, President Reagan was quoted as saying, "Trees cause more pollution than automobiles do." As satire, the Swarthmore contingent created a large cardboard placard, with a tree painted on it, which read: CHOP ME DOWN BEFORE I KILL AGAIN. It was handed to me to brandish.

As we entered the main plaza, where the oration was to occur, two Secret Service Neanderthals, who made Bruno and Rufus look like wimps in comparison, grabbed me roughly and started dragging me away from the protest. They escorted me through their ranks to a back entrance, so that the other Swarthmore students couldn't follow.

They gravely accused me of "threatening the president" but were otherwise silent as we walked away from the crowd. They ignored my requests to see their badges, and my explanations about the meaning of my sign. Eventually, we arrived at their car, they searched my pockets, and our discussion began in earnest.

"Are you a student?"
"Yes, at Swarthmore."

"What are you doing out here today?"

"Protesting President Reagan's visit."

"Do you know that your sign is threatening?"

"To who???"

"The president. You are threatening to 'kill again.'"

"The tree is threatening to 'kill again.' President Reagan says that trees cause more pollution than cars. Pollution kills people."

"The sign says, 'Chop me down before I kill again.'"

"It's the tree speaking. It's satire. It's conceptual, sort of like a metaphor. The 'chop me down' refers to the tree depicted on the poster, sort of daring President Reagan to chop it down, because, according to him, trees kill people."

"Have you ever been arrested?"

"No."

"Charged with any crimes?"

"No."

"In prison?"

"Why would you go to prison without being arrested or charged with any crimes?"

"Why do you have more than one ID on you?"

"All teenagers do this to get into concerts."

"What is your favorite drug?"

"Coffee."

"This is not a joke. What is your drug of choice?"

"If you are offering, coffee with milk and one Equal. I would never do any other drugs. They are illegal."

"We can give you your sign back, and then we might have to arrest you, or we can confiscate the sign and let you go."

"Why don't you keep the sign. It's more trouble than it's worth."

As they were finally letting me go, a group of twenty Swarthmore students, who had been frantically looking for me, caught up with us and started yelling "Fascist pigs!" Having just extricated myself, I energetically waved them off. Enough drama for one day.

Back on campus, I enjoyed my celebrity status. "Oh, *you're* the guy that got shaken down by Reagan's thugs?" This notoriety nudged me toward a more drug-experimenting set of friends, more leftist and nonconformist. I decided to be a philosophy major and to take my premed courses on the side.

Having lost my rehab Waterloo, I was too busy to mope or to fret. The positive test for Valium started a chain reaction of excruciating consequences.

I was required back in court, as usual, at 8:00 the next morning. The agreement that we had come up with just a month previously, which gave me a long leash, was violated by this positive test. When we went back, I faced a less sympathetic judge, more of a typical white, male, middle-aged, overweight, balding, mainstream, druggie-hating, Republican kind of judge.

Solomon was busy that day, so I was represented by his understudy, Eric, who was young, mild-mannered, and bespectacled. He looked like a teenager. He didn't fill me with confidence. I never thought I'd miss Solomon's insulting personality.

Eric kept leaving my side and, just out of earshot, engaged in frenzied, contentious consultations with the district attorney. The judge insisted I return in two weeks' time for sentencing. Eric said I couldn't, because I'd be in rehab. The judge finally assented to a date four months later, provided that I had spent at least three of those months in rehab. The vibe in the courtroom had changed from "Good luck with your recovery, Doctor" to "If you screw up again, you will pay dearly." I was in a different ontological category.

As negotiated by Solomon, I was placed on medical leave from my academic position at the hospital. This was better than being fired, which they did anyway a few months later. I discussed my medical leave at an interview with the medical director of the Faulkner Hospital, Dr. John. Ever since he was my attending on the medical service, as a resident, I had worshipped him as an empathic and talented physician. Now I felt like I had let him down personally.

"Dr. John, I really appreciate all that you've done for me. My situation with the board is serious. The criminal charges are serious. I don't know when I'll be able to work again, but I hope we'll have a chance to work together again. I'll turn this around."

After listening patiently to my speech, he stood up, came around his desk, and gave me a hug. Awkward as it was, a middle-aged doctor hugging a fallen colleague, I will never forget how validated and understood I felt, even if only for that brief moment. It was the first time since before Bruno and Rufus came into my office that anyone not related to me by blood or on my immediate caregiving team treated me like a human being. Many of the others were treating me like I was radioactive and contagious.

That night, after putting the kids to sleep, I drove back to my office, late enough so that I was unlikely to have an embarrassing, chance interaction with anyone, trying to find some peace of mind and organize some papers. My brain was sizzling with paranoia about rehab.

I had agreed not to "practice medicine," which I interpreted as not conducting any more patient visits, though no one actually spelled out what it meant. Surely I could clean up some of the mess I was leaving for my colleagues, and at least organize my desk for the day I would be allowed to return to my job. I was still viewing all of this as a brief interruption.

I had often gone to my office in the evenings after the kids were put to bed, under the pretext of having work to finish but really as a way to avoid my worsening marriage. On these nights, I went to my office with the best of intentions, planning to catch up on labs and send letters out to patients. But it was rare that I didn't have a stash in my bag, or in my desk, which would slowly start murmuring to me.

I would try crushing, chopping up, and snorting Oxycontin, but this was never very effective. I am a mouth breather and have chronic allergies, so very little entered my bloodstream via my nose, and I mostly ended up looking like a drunk prostitute who had just put on a messy coat of white makeup. The powder tasted bitter, and it would drip down from my nose into my throat for hours.

On this particular evening, the key to my office just wouldn't work, no matter how much I jiggled and jimmied. This had never happened before. It was a simple lock that always had popped right open. From the hallway, through the glass windows, I could see into the waiting room, with the neatened stacks of magazines, the antismoking posters, and the still-cluttered reception desk, geared up for action the next day.

After fumbling with the keys for a few minutes, I started to get irritated and vaguely unsettled. With all I had been through the last few weeks, I didn't need this minor, random obstacle. All I wanted was some peace and quiet, and to get some work done. After about five more minutes of increasingly frenetic attempts on the lock, and several fantasies about smashing through the window and unlocking the door from inside, I called security for assistance.

I'd known the security officer, Billy, since my first day on the job several years earlier, an amiable Irish American with whom I had always joked or at least exchanged pleasantries. He was a patient of our practice, so I had cared for him during cross coverage. We had an easy rapport. He took a long time to arrive, looked uncomfortable and embarrassed, even apologetic, and stated, "I'm sorry, Dr. Grinspoon, the locks have been changed and I've been instructed not to let you in."

I heard these words, but they were so unexpected, and so foreign, that I couldn't process them. Like someone afflicted with Broca's brain, I couldn't speak.

"Billy, ummm, what???"

"I can't let you in. I'm sorry."

(*Heated*) "Who is telling you not to let me in?"

"Dr. Grinspoon, please, I'm just doing my job."

"Yes, of course. I'm sorry. Thanks for coming up. It's nice to see you. Take care of yourself."

Locked out of my office? I was only on medical leave. Why would they do this? There hadn't been a single patient complaint about me. This felt like a colossal betrayal. I had counted on my colleagues being supportive. I considered these colleagues to be my friends. We freely joked together, asked each other for clinical advice, and even socialized together. What's a few criminal charges among friends?

Then it hit me. No one was going to let me back into the office again. This was over, because I had screwed it up. I was being stripped of my medical license and my privileges at this hospital. I was in the process of being dropped by all of the HMOs and insurance plans that I participated in, and of losing my board certification in internal medicine. This was no longer some mild scrape that I could talk myself out of. It was something larger that I had better wake up and start paying attention to, immediately.

The summer after my first year at Swarthmore, Martin and I, accompanied by Jason, a brilliant philosophy major from Montana, and a few other friends, spent the summer in Berkeley, California. I took courses in rhetoric and classical literature. We lived in one of the student-run co-ops.

We went to several concerts at Berkeley's Greek Theatre, a beautiful and storied outdoor venue. During one concert at the Greek, we were smoking cannabis openly like most people. Safety in numbers. Nearby, we saw a young concertgoer, dressed much like us, scruffy, in shorts and T-shirt, speaking earnestly, almost conspiratorially, with a uniformed police officer. There was something about this conversation that caught our interest, possibly the knowing, furtive glances he sent our way.

As we watched, he left the police officer, took a deliberately circuitous route around sections of the crowd, and then casually approached us. He tried to employ a groovy, freewheeling, stoner shuffle, which made him look like he had Parkinson's disease.

> *"Hey, man. Great concert! How's it going?"*
> "Good, thanks."
> *"Can I buy some of that stuff you're smoking?"*
> "What?"
> *"Can I buy some weed from you?"*
> "What are you talking about?"

"I want to buy some weed. I saw you smoking some earlier."

"There are twenty thousand people here smoking. Why on earth are you asking us?"

"I know you have some, I saw you smoking it, and I really just want to buy a little. Just enough to catch a buzz, help me enjoy the concert. Please? I'd really appreciate it."

At that point, he pulled out some crumpled bills and tried to foist them on us. He was really insistent, almost aggressive. Given that we were high and, as he suspected, we were in possession, we decided to get rid of him as quickly as possible, not to have fun by tormenting him.

Jason, holding up a bag of tobacco, which, fortuitously, he had with him, yelled, *"It's tobacco!* We were smoking home-rolled cigarettes, that's all. I'm sorry we can't hook you up." This undercover cop fell out of character, turned, and, businesslike, with a slightly martial gait, walked away without a word and rejoined his uniformed colleague.

Having forgotten, or put out of my mind, the nightmare that Will went through when he dropped acid with us in high school, I decided to try LSD again, this time at a Grateful Dead concert. A friend of Jason's had just mailed him some, and this small blotter of colored paper was getting restless sitting in Jason's bedside drawer.

The effect started subtly. When I turned my head, the image of the previous object I was looking at lingered on and became superimposed onto the image of the next thing in my field of vision. Whooaah. Then the previous image would slowly fade, like the bright spot behind the eyelids after a camera flash. I also noted that the lovely fragrance of the sycamore trees bypassed my nose and wafted directly into my brain stem.

Joyously wandering around the streets of Berkeley, I eventually made my way into the concert, past some brief paranoia when they collected my ticket. One of the guards at the concert said to me, "Berkeley, California. Planet Earth. Nineteen eighty-five." It was a good guess that any particular concertgoer could use some orientation. I thanked him and marveled at how he could possibly know so much and be so self-assured.

I was absolutely euphoric until the end of the concert, when the Dead played a cover of Bob Dylan's "It's All Over Now, Baby Blue." The mournfulness of this song caused me to start to despair. My emotional reactions were becoming exaggerated.

The sun was setting, and this affected me viscerally. I was feeling very alone, and the world started becoming sinister in a way that only LSD can trigger The very substance of the world, the molecules themselves, in some indefinable way, were somehow wrong and no longer friendly. I wandered out when the concert ended and sat down heavily on the first bench I could find.

Next to me, a group of Deadheads were juggling bowling pins that were flaming on one end. This was giving me vertigo, especially because the area where the flame had been stayed lit up for more than a few seconds. The brightness of the flames was making the rest of the world appear even darker.

People were drumming and chanting, and I felt less and less connected to this cultural reality. I must have looked distraught. Just as I was losing hope, through the noise and commotion I heard, "Grinspoon, where the *fuck* have you been? What are you doing here? You look like crap." Four hours after we had separated, my friends caught up with me. Knowing that I was tripping, they were looking for me. Jason stayed up with me for hours, strumming on his guitar, grinning at the nonsense I was spouting, which I thought was absolutely brilliant.

During this episode, I caught a glimpse, even more personal and vivid than what I witnessed through Will's meltdown, of how drugs can have an exceedingly dark, destructive side. From then on, I avoided LSD like a plague, and likely would have avoided hallucinogens altogether, if it weren't for my family's friendship with Sasha Shulgin.

A few weeks later, I saw a copy of a letter sent to my patients, informing them that I was no longer at Primary Care Internal

Medicine Associates, which was the first news I received that they wouldn't be holding my job for me.

Between the courts, the police, Society to Help Physicians, the board, and my guilt and shame, I hadn't had the time, or the courage, to sit down and discuss what had happened with the other docs in my practice. Given the daily worsening of my position, it would have been difficult to keep my colleagues updated, like a floor trader trying to keep his bosses apprised of share prices during Black Thursday.

Out of dire necessity, to explain the obvious, and to avoid burning bridges, I had gathered the courage to make an appointment with my medical director, Dr. Hutch. Dr. Hutch is tall and neat-appearing, with longish hair, a throwback to distant hippie times. He is friendly and well-intentioned, if somewhat narcissistic and stubborn. He has always been quick to laugh, but also quick to criticize the clinical decisions of the other doctors in the practice. He was a friend that I was slightly wary of.

His office was lined with pictures of his successful children, one of whom was about to go to Yale. At that point, I wasn't sure that Annie and Milo were going to make it to the end of elementary school. I explained the chronology and depth of what was happening; I owed him at least that. I assured him that I hadn't been impaired at work. Shaking his head, he solemnly replied, "There I go, by God!" He, like me, is Jewish, and I think he meant to say "There but for the grace of God go I."

When I look back upon this period, it is no wonder that the hospital administration, and even my colleagues, would take an aggressively conservative position. I was out of control, and they had every reason to be concerned about my having unfettered access to the prescription samples closet, or to other people's prescription pads. Addicts, myself included, are scary and they steal. They are nothing but trouble. Especially from the vantage point of clean-cut doctors with kids to support and careers to nourish. Any uncertainty or danger is to be avoided.

But locking me out of the office without telling me? At that point I was so far from viewing myself as a danger or a threat, or a criminal, or an outlaw, or anything but the nice, friendly doctor that I still believed myself to be, that I simply couldn't comprehend why they would change the locks. Deeply shaken, with nowhere else to go, I drove back home, convinced that my life couldn't possibly get any worse.

Driving as slowly as possible, I considered what to share with H., and how thoroughly I should update her on the situation. H. knew about the criminal charges and the agreement not to practice medicine, and I couldn't really hide the fact that I was already spending big money on legal fees. She would probably notice my upcoming absence at rehab for three months. As I was starting to have vague forebodings about our future, I wasn't sure she needed to know anything else.

Sasha Shulgin, known as the Godfather of Psychedelics, was a Berkeley biochemist who created different designer drugs with varying psychedelic properties. He was just another bad-news friend of the Grinspoon family.

On several occasions, I tried an experimental psychedelic called 2CB, which Sasha designed. The experience was invariably gentle, relaxing, euphoric, and interesting. It had none of the nightmare qualities of acid, and I was left with a crystal-clear memory of what I had hallucinated. Who knows how it worked, or what it did to my brain.

As my summer in Berkeley was ending, I had to scramble to study for my exams, having been uncharacteristically lax due to the multifarious distractions in Berkeley. A fellow student offered me some Benzedrine, a powerful amphetamine, to help me study. I didn't know at the time that this was the loaded gun known as methamphetamine, which is currently ruining so many lives.

On the Benzedrine, I had never been so alert or so productive. I absorbed the Cliff's Notes on the classics I was supposed to have read at an astonishing pace, retained the knowledge with crystal clarity, and aced the exam. Afterward, I felt more contaminated from using Cliff's Notes than from using meth. I was brought up to believe that using Cliff's Notes was wrong.

I was too preoccupied with my woes to notice that H. was waiting for me on the front porch, sitting in the dark with the front door open. It was fairly late into the evening, and I expected that the kids were both asleep. It was too dark for me to see her facial expression, or I might have been stopped in my tracks. I didn't notice that she was shaking and crying.

"Hi, H., what are you doing out here? Aren't you cold?"
"*Get out. Don't come any closer. Don't come into my house. Don't come near my kids. You don't live here anymore. Go stay with your parents.*"

Unable to advance, or to leave, I sat down on the front walk. She pulled something small out of her pocket and flung it at me with all of her might. "Take these with you." And then she slammed the door.

What did she throw? Manna from heaven? Pills? Is she trying to get me to overdose?

Numb, out of ideas, and curious as to what she had thrown at me, I started crawling around the front lawn, using the faint light of my cell phone to illuminate my search. It had rained the night before, and I could feel my knees getting moist and cold through my jeans, as they sank into the mud. On the edge of the circular patch of dirt from which a giant dogwood was growing, which we planted when Annie was born, I found one of a pair of small gold earrings, a family heirloom that my mother had given her, welcoming her into the family as a new daughter. Ouch. This was even worse than pills. She wasn't just trying to bump me off, but was truly trying to sever ties.

I sat in my car until I saw our bedroom light go off. I felt like I was watching a tragic movie of someone else's life. Waiting another thirty minutes so that H. would be sound asleep, I quietly went in and gathered some bare essentials. At least these locks hadn't been changed, or it would have been twice in one evening that I was locked out.

I went to stay with my parents, who still lived in my childhood home, about twenty minutes away. They weren't particularly surprised to see me, and my possessions, showing up at midnight. They knew there had been trouble in paradise for quite some time.

My parents were aware, factually, about my addiction, but I don't think they fully understood how much distress I was in. It was hard for them to discern what was what in my rapidly deteriorating life, with my broken marriage, my job that had just gone poof, and the drugs they suspected I was taking. They would take me in no matter what I had done.

"You're back," said my dad. "Take off your shoes before walking on the carpet with your things."

"Are you hungry? Can I feed you anything?" was my mom's response. Fortunately, neither of them alluded to the drugs, or the marital meltdown, which I wasn't ready to talk about. I already missed my kids and it had been all of thirty minutes.

My father is a prominent psychiatrist who, in a cosmic irony, happens to specialize in substances of abuse. It must have been particularly difficult for him to sense that I might be suffering from one of the deadly addictive syndromes he had written about so eloquently. Having *his son* suffer from addiction was out of his frame of reference, and he didn't know what to say.

My mom just felt bad for me and supported me as much as she could under the circumstances. She is one of those unconditionally nurturing people who would welcome back Jeffrey Dahmer or Benito Mussolini and ask them what she could do for them. Addiction was entirely foreign to her.

Both of my parents were quite worried about Annie and Milo and the turbulence they must have been experiencing.

There was nothing left for me to do but to read books and count down the remaining days until rehab. At that point, it felt as if everything was being stripped away from me. H. allowed me a brief good-bye with Annie and Milo the day before my departure. We all cried, and I had to pry their hands off me when I left. She later accused me of being high during this visit.

Trying to cheer me up with some levity, my twin brother started referring to my upcoming tenure at rehab as my "extreme makeover." "Did your extreme makeover start yet? Are you looking forward to the extreme makeover? How's the extreme makeover going?" He gave me books by Carl Hiaasen (*Skinny Dip*) and Jonathan Franzen (*The Corrections*) to help pass the time.

Under this false cheer, my twin was extremely worried about me. We were as close as two brothers could be, as if we hadn't fully separated at birth. I had forgiven him for ditching me in the hospital just after we were born. He saw what mayhem my life was descending into, but it was entirely beyond his experience and he didn't really know how to help. "Peter, you've really got to get this together. Do whatever it takes."

My older brother, David, was more savvy, having had a wife who struggled with her drinking. He gave me an iPod with thousands of songs, so I could blot out the religious chatter I was about to be bombarded with for the next twelve weeks.

PART TWO

Extreme Makeover

During the long trip to North Carolina, I drove slowly, out of sheer dread of arriving. I even meandered through the toxic wastelands of New Jersey, recirculating the air so I wouldn't asphyxiate. The cars behind me were blaring their horns to hurry me along, with increasing stridency the farther south I was. I could imagine them thinking "Goddamn carpetbagger Yankee slowpoke dipshit."

As I drove, I listened to the song "Karma" by the Black Eyed Peas, over and over again, with its mesmeric refrain, "Ain't no runnin' from Karma...It's gonna get ya, yeah, yeah, yeah." These lyrics encapsulated my predicament in a nutshell. I was convinced that I must have been incarnated as something really bad in a previous life to deserve this. Attila the Hun? Caligula? I brushed that thought away; I already had enough to feel guilty about.

It felt disorienting, to say the least, to be driving away from my job, patients, kids, wife, friends, cousins, and possessions, not knowing which of these, if any, would be waiting for me upon my return, or who I would be at that point.

On the interstate, just over the Virginia border, a large blue sign said, **DRUG** CHECKPOINT FOUR MILES. Finally, a word that my brain could relate to, to rouse me out of my depressed stupor. At this point in my life, whenever I so much as entered a CVS and went back to the pharmacy counter, the labels of the controlled substances would glow and dance in front of my eyes in hallucinatory gestures of beckoning.

Out of deeply ingrained instinct, and because I usually had at least marijuana in the car, I almost veered off onto the one obscure exit that presented itself to me before the four miles were up. This exit led to a very small town, without an obvious gas station or other amenities at its departure point from the highway. I suddenly remembered a previous (cannabis-induced) insight: If I act innocent, my crime remains invisible. I elected to remain on the highway, surmising that they couldn't possibly stop every car.

As I drove by, I noticed, at the bottom of this exit ramp, a large gathering of state troopers and drug units. A trap. Sneaky motherfuckers. If you turned onto this exit, you almost certainly had drugs in your car. You drove right into their hands. They picked an exit that practically no one would plausibly visit.

Even though I wasn't carrying anything, it would have been time-consuming and humiliating to convince these (redneck fascist) Virginia state troopers of my innocence. "Really, officer, I'm a doctor who *used* to be on drugs, but I'm not now, and I only took this exit out of preservation instinct. I'm driving from Boston down to rehab in North Carolina." Good luck with that story. And what if there were still some pills or traces of reefer in my car that I had forgotten about and that their drug hounds sniffed out? I wouldn't have even made it to rehab.

The next day, I finally reached Tannenberg Rehab. I couldn't believe how many pancake and waffle houses there were lining the main drag of the local town. This must be how the citizens of North Carolina keep so trim and healthy. From Harvard Medical to Waffle Hell. What next? I shuddered to think where this trajectory would lead.

I spent my last night of freedom restlessly roaming this tacky wasteland. The whole town was one big Christmas Tree Shop. I thought about getting drunk as a last act of rebellion, but then I remembered that I didn't like alcohol because it made me feel itchy and restless.

I settled for gorging on comfort food from Taco Hell and sleeping in a bare-bones, musty Econo Lodge, which had stains on the carpet, mold in the sink, and enough dust to trigger my asthma.

Watching *The Bourne Supremacy* on TV, I swallowed a small handful of my remaining Klonapin and dozed into anxious dreams of a medieval, cloistered place called rehab, which, in this dream, was strangely peopled with my family and acquaintances. The last two things I scribbled in my diary before drifting off, handwriting blurrier as the Klonapin kicked in, were "what did I do to my life?" and "what is my life doing to me?"

One night, before my biology final at Swarthmore, I absolutely couldn't fall asleep. The rain pattering on the window was jangling my nerves. With each minute, I was more worried that, if I didn't fall asleep right away, I wouldn't do well on my final and wouldn't get into med school. This thinking precluded sleep.

Increasingly worried, I started to have a panic attack, with racing heart and thoughts, a feeling that wouldn't be recreated for twenty years until, at Tannenberg Rehab, I was taken off my Klonapin. I couldn't wake any of my friends for help, because they had exams the next morning as well, and besides, I wouldn't know what to say to them.

At about 2:00 in the morning, in a desperate burst of impulsiveness, I ran over to my psychiatrist Dr. Surgeon's house, about ten minutes away in the sleepy village of Swarthmore. I was so intent on reaching his house immediately, once I decided to go there, that I didn't even put shoes on and ran barefoot in the rain, which was exhilarating after lying in a stifling bed for several hours, worrying myself to death and unable to sleep.

Dr. Surgeon, after his initial shock and concern from being awoken at 2:00 a.m., ascertained that, wet, muddy, and bedraggled as I was, I was not a home invader. Instead of telling me to go away, or to go to the hospital, he invited me into his office and conversed with me for at least an hour until I calmed down. This moved me deeply and, on some level, reinforced my desire to become a physician, so that I could be as empathic and life-sustaining as Dr. Surgeon was to me that night.

At Swarthmore, I was having worsening insomnia and, for my worsening anxiety, I had started seeing a psychiatrist. I knew I needed help, because I was developing a compulsive inner dialogue about my perceived failures. "You should study harder. Why didn't you get a better grade on that test? Why are you wasting time trying to be a doctor?" My diary from the time is scribbled full of these thoughts.

The main issue I worked on with Dr. Surgeon was convincing myself that I was worthy of being loved by other people. Some of this fear stemmed from Danny's death and lack of emotional constancy. Some of it was neurotic. With Dr. Surgeon's help, I managed to remain relatively even-keeled.

Dr. Surgeon also helped me figure out what to do with myself after college. While I had already invested countless exceedingly dry and brainless hours as a premed, there was no way I was mature enough or interested enough to go straight from college to medical school.

Maybe I was still reacting to the injustice of a world where the Secret Service could drag you away with no warning. Or possibly I was responding to the rhetoric in my left-wing philosophy seminars about how we need to take responsibility for the world. Maybe my childhood exposures to the Famous Astronomers and Poets of the world had inspired me more than they seemed to at the time. Or perhaps it was just too much fun to outsmart undercover policemen in Berkeley.

Milking a family connection, I was hired as an administrative assistant to Greenpeace's Nuclear Free Seas campaign.

Back in the Econo Lodge, I woke up in a stupor the next morning, not solely from the Klonapin, or the asthma, but from the combined metabolic effect of every molecule in my body wishing to avoid starting the next ninety days. For the first time in my life, I couldn't think of a single thing to look forward to. I drew a blank. Work? Kids? Wife? Upcoming vacations? Paycheck? Sex? No, no, and no. Drugs? Definitely no. At 8:00 a.m., after—what else?—a waffle breakfast, I dragged myself over the threshold into rehab, into what I was absolutely convinced was going to be the First Circle of Hell.

Tannenberg Rehab is located in an old inn on five acres of land. The thick air smelled sweet, like ripe vegetation and tobacco smoke. The sunlight was filtering through a dense canopy of trees, creating the illusion of an oasis of peacefulness, shimmering and dancing in stark contrast to the terror I felt as I climbed up the front steps.

Bedraggled as I looked, unshowered, unshaven, frumpily dressed, and with Klonapin eyes, no one seemed to notice my arrival. Partially, this was because I had stumbled upon the dominant fashion trend in rehab, and I blended right in. Good thing I left the tuxedo at home. I saw my reflection in the glass of the front door and noticed that I had put my shirt on inside out. This made me look like a mental patient, but I was too nervous and preoccupied to be overly self-conscious.

As I paced back and forth, waiting for the staff to notice me, I heard a murmur of voices and laughter coming from a fenced-in area to the left of the main entrance. Sneaking up to observe, I saw groups of patients congregated in the gardens, smoking, joking, and laughing. I immediately sensed a different vibe from the Talbott Center, where the inmates seemed so morbidly hopeless and apathetic.

In contrast, the vibe at Tannenberg felt more like a gang of naughty teenagers in detention, busted for doing something fun but contraband, killing time together. This offered me a speck of hope, amid generalized despair.

Tannenberg treated many doctors and nurses, but there were also many coal miners from Kentucky, who were victims of the Appalachian Oxycontin epidemic. I think that their tuition was subsidized; otherwise, it would cost them a year of salary to stay at Tannenberg for a month. I came from the heights of Harvard Medical, and they came from the darkest depths of the coal pits, but we were brought to the same place by the same drug. There were also teachers trying to sober up during their summer break, as well as lawyers, businessmen, housewives, and laborers.

The patients seemed evenly split between drugs and alcohol. The alcoholics disdained the drug addicts because their disease was more socially acceptable.

There were trust-fund hippies, who generally had very few brain cells left and who tended to stare off into space most of the time. They seemed like empty shadows. Always the anthropologist, I indulgently speculated that their pitiable state was because they didn't have any occupation or identity to revert to if and when they overcame their addiction.

"Hi, Dr. Grinspoon, I'm Jasmin, the chief nurse." I jumped. Why did she have to sneak up behind me? Is that part of the treatment?

"Can you please empty your pockets so that I can search you?"

"What???"

I was being treated like a criminal by a plump, middle-aged nurse. This started collapsing my sense of self. Evenly, she continued, "People try to smuggle things in here all the time. We've had people try to drink hair spray and nail polish remover. We need to search your bag as well."

I swore up and down that I didn't have any nail polish remover stashed away. "While you are here, please watch your possessions carefully, because this place is full of drug addicts." Drug addicts in rehab? You don't say.

After exhaustively patting me down, Jasmin said it was time to go through my car. The Fates seemed determined to have my car searched, if not by the Virginia police, waiting in their Venus flytrap, then by Jasmin.

Jasmin was joined by another nurse, who must have been seven feet tall, blonde, cold as ice, and who carried the moniker "The Amazon." They went through every crevice of my car, including under the seats. I was indignant at the thoroughness of their search, until they started excavating in the trunk, under where the spare tire was kept. They hit pay dirt. Jasmin said, "I knew it," in a tone one might use when scolding a three-year-old who had soiled his Pull-Up.

I had packed bottles of Tylenol, Advil, Sudafed, Benadryl, Excedrin, Robitussin, Pepto-Bismol, and Zantac, so that I would be comfortable and have some control over my withdrawal symptoms. When they started removing these bottles, I lodged a vigorous protest. These were not controlled or abusable substances.

Anyone can buy them at any pharmacy, and there was no reason to confiscate them.

My protest fell on deaf ears. The detox process, when the staff transition patients off the drug they were taking up until their arrival, is medically dangerous. The staff need to carefully control all medicines, even the over-the-counter meds, so they can readily assess and treat any physical problems, such as swings in blood pressure. This process can take weeks, depending on what you are addicted to. Patients definitely weren't allowed to self-medicate. Especially doctors. That's how we got here in the first place.

What Jasmin and the Amazon weren't hearing was that these were my comfort objects, which I brought with me to soothe me through the upcoming dark times. These were my teddy bear and my favorite blanket. Now I had to face this alone and trust these strangers to manage my withdrawal symptoms. It felt odd to be a doctor who wasn't even allowed to take his own Tylenol. I had really come down in the world.

From my car, I was next led to the nurses' station, for the next phase of my intake. I was starting to feel, again, like I was on a different planet.

The nurses at Tannenberg were really working me over.

"Sit down here. We're going to take your vital signs. How are you feeling?"

"I'm feeling like I want you to give those bottles of medicine back."

"We're going to take your vital signs every few hours for the next several days to make sure you aren't having any dangerous withdrawal symptoms. Can you please blow into this tube?"

What??? Now I'm supposed to give a plastic tube a blow job? This was getting worse and worse.

"It's a breathalyzer test to measure your alcohol level. After this, it's time for your first drug test."

After blowing, I was escorted to the laboratory and medication room, which was secured by the fastened lower half of a split door. The top half of the door was open, and I could see several nurses filling the locked boxes, which contained the medications that the other residents were taking. I noticed a small mountain of urine specimen kits.

They unlocked the door, let me through, and quickly locked it again. I didn't understand this defensive arrangement. If someone wanted to, they could leap into the room by catapulting over the locked bottom half of the door.

On the far side of this room was an open urinal, without any privacy, where I was asked to provide a specimen. It's a good thing I don't have a shy bladder, because I was being observed by what seemed to me at the time to be menacing, psychosexually starved nurses, who were watching my every move with eagle eyes lest I attempt to tamper with the specimen.

At long last, they took me to what was going to be my room for the first two weeks of my twelve-week stay, until I demonstrated enough medical stability and mature behavior to "graduate" to the off-campus housing. I was emotionally drained from the intake, and still reeling from the way they treated me like a convict. I was spent, and no longer had the fortitude to engage in complex interactions. I was finally looking forward to some peace and quiet.

In 1991, I was invited to Kiev as part of an international team, spearheaded by Greenpeace, to organize publicity around the fifth anniversary of the reactor disaster at Chernobyl. Just to get to these reactors, we had to drive through an enormous abandoned zone, thirty kilometers in diameter. It reminded me of the "Forbidden Zone" in *Planet of the Apes*, except that it had trees and grass, and was full of animals.

Our first stop was the control room of the reactor. As if this whole thing were a spoof, they gave us white cloth caps to protect us from any radiation spills. These flimsy hats had side flaps that drooped down my neck like bunny ears. They were worn by all the employees at the reactor, giving the whole place a surreal, comical atmosphere. It was as if kindergarteners were putting on a play about running a nuclear reactor.

The control room for the reactors looked as shabby as the rest of Ukraine, like some run-down set from a B-rated 1950s science fiction movie. There was trash on the floor. There were large arrays of flashing lights and controls, many of them with broken bulbs. The people manning these control panels seemed about as alert as Homer Simpson, who would have been disappointed working there, eating beets instead of doughnuts. He probably would have emigrated and tried to claim asylum.

After a banquet of beets and vodka, and after suffering through the increasingly drunken speeches, we were allowed to tour the rest of the plant and to come to within a few kilometers of the exploded reactor, which loomed in the distance, a hulking concrete sarcophagus. As my Geiger counter went berserk, I thought anxiously of my private parts and my future, unborn children. To minimize exposure, we stayed there for only a little while, and we all wore extra pairs of underwear.

Staring at this enormous radioactive concrete mass, the cause of so many deaths, so many cancers, so much turmoil, and so much abandoned territory, I realized on a deep level that humans really could poison themselves out of existence if we didn't, as a species, mend our ways quickly.

After touring the ghost town of Pripyat, we met with citizens' groups in the communal areas of dilapidated Soviet-era apartment buildings, where every conceivable ailment was blamed on the radiation, even twisted ankles and AIDS. The whole community seemed to have given up hope. I can imagine the level of learned helplessness, when a nuclear reactor blows up near you and the government is incompetent at best, and spreads disinformation.

We visited farmers whose fields were radioactive and who were required to rotate their farm animals to distant farms, so that they would graze on the contaminated land for only a short part of their lifespan. The authorities decided that it was better to have most animals somewhat radioactive than to have some animals highly radioactive. I guess they needed the meat. At that point, having eaten only beets since my arrival, I would have gobbled down any meat, regardless of protests from my Geiger counter.

We toured a children's hospital, which was sparsely stocked with broken-down equipment and expired medications sent from relief agencies in Europe. I picked up a vial of penicillin that had expired five years earlier. These young kids with thyroid cancer and leukemia deserved better than this. Of course, my brother Danny had the absolute best of everything, and he still died.

I felt particularly linked to the antinuclear protests at Greenpeace because of my brother Danny's death. When my parents lived in California, in the late 1950s, Danny, like many other children, was exposed to low-level radioactive fallout from the above-ground nuclear testing that was still being practiced by our government. My parents gave Danny and David canned milk to drink in order to minimize radiation exposure. The radiation they couldn't avoid might have contributed to his leukemia in the first place, which got my entire family smoking pot.

Now, at Greenpeace, I was trying to help protect other kids from a similar kind of radioactive exposure.

In addition to providing me with a sense of unity and purpose, Greenpeace placed me at an epicenter of the Just Say No era's drug culture. I attended private rooftop parties with members of the Grateful Dead and other luminaries of the left. I went to elite countercultural gatherings at our headquarters in Amsterdam, where hashish and other drugs are legal, as well as events in London, Paris, and Dublin.

The environment we were protecting was saturated in recreational drugs, which reinforced my drug-taking behaviors. For the five years I was at Greenpeace, like the preceding four in college, the message I received about drugs was that they were a positive adjunct to all of the fun things going on. At some point, this type of message starts to sink in.

I studied for the Medical College Admission Test (MCAT) through clouds of smoke and blaring Grateful Dead bootlegs, bumping up and down in the back of the Greenpeace van en route to civil disobedience actions. The lyrics to "Uncle John's

Band" blended in my mind with the organic reactions I was studying. Come hear methyl ethyl ketone, reacting with the tide. I would carefully stash my textbooks under the seat as we got out to protest, so I would know where to reclaim them later if we were arrested. I studied on Greenpeace ships until I was so seasick that I had to put my textbooks away.

If only, during the actual MCAT, they had pumped in marijuana smoke, piped in the Grateful Dead, had my seat bumping and rolling, and interrupted the test periodically to put me in handcuffs, I likely would have received a perfect score and been accepted to Harvard Medical.

I had also studied for the MCAT in Kiev, on the bus, driving around Chernobyl. If there were an award, or extra credit, for the most radioactive textbook in the United States, I would have won it hands down upon my return.

At Greenpeace, there was no negative feedback for breaking the law. With this type of subversive thinking deeply ingrained in my early twenties, it became easier to rationalize a variety of unethical behaviors. This proved critical in creating the frame of mind where a doctor and an addict could coexist. It enabled lines to be crossed. Many of the skills I honed in the role of a guerrilla activist at Greenpeace, such as stealing, stealth, and deception, later helped me sustain my addiction.

The door to my room in Tannenberg opened to twin beds on either side of the doorway, with spare furniture, a well-worn rug, and fluorescent lights, a cross between a dorm room and a cheap hotel. The room was occupied by a thick-haired, portly, disheveled man, seemingly in his midthirties, of medium height, who was pacing, and bellowing to himself in a dense southern accent: "They're tryin' to kill me; they're fuckin' tryin' to kill me."

He didn't acknowledge my presence or even notice that I had entered this small room. My "Hello, I'm Peter Grinspoon" echoed and faded into the sound of his muttering and his footsteps without evoking a response. He ignored my outstretched hand.

Exhausted from the degrading conveyor belt I had just ridden, and from the novelty of being an inmate, I put down my bags, lay on my bed, and despite my roommate's angry monologue, I soon became lost in the utter dysfunctionality of the Lambert family in *The Corrections* by Jonathan Franzen.

It made me feel better to read about these fictional characters with their fictional problems. It distracted me from the fact that I was reeling inside from my transition to this new and strange world. I just couldn't come to believe that I was stuck here for ninety days, removed from everyone and everything that I cared about. I was surrounded by complete strangers. We were united only in our overindulgence in either drugs or drink. The drugged-out loser fuckup club. How depressing!

Eventually, my roommate's pacing slowed, the bellowing quieted, and abruptly he turned to me, with genuine puzzlement in his cloudy red eyes, and asked, "Where'd you come from?"

This was my roommate, Lyle. He had been awake since his arrival two days earlier, and was caught up in a temporary insanity that resulted from the abrupt cessation of Oxycontin combined with the heavy medication cocktail the nurses had given him to steer him back toward Earth. He had concluded that the nurses were trying to poison him.

After a few minutes of explanation, Lyle understood that, having just arrived, I was entirely innocent of the plot to poison him. Desperate to bond with someone, and forgetting that I was in the South, I further introduced myself by way of complaining about how religious the program seemed.

"Why is everyone so obsessed with God around here? They've all been brainwashed. How can God cure a disease? Why would he create the disease in the first place?"

Lyle looked puzzled. These statements were outside of his immediate frame of reference, so it ground our conversation to a halt.

When it eventually resumed, I learned that Lyle had recently been arrested for criminal possession of methadone (a drug similar to Oxycontin) at his solo dental practice. The state police almost caught him with Oxycontin as well, but he locked himself in the private bathroom of his office and snorted and flushed all of it, with the officers pounding on the door outside.

Lyle lives in a small town in the rural South, and his arrest made the front page of the local newspaper for the reading pleasure of his family, friends, patients, and any small-town gossipmongers. Lyle had spent all of his money on drugs; even his car was repossessed. His dental license was suspended.

As Lyle described it, the police in the rural South aren't particularly enlightened about addiction. Nor are they warm and fuzzy. They pressured Lyle to wear a wire and to then solicit Oxycontin from his dealer, hoping to record the conversation and bust his dealer in the act. Their threats and promises reminded me of my dealings with Bruno and Rufus: coerced cooperation bartered for vague promises of leniency.

Lyle told them, "Hell no, you all are gonna get me killed." He refused them, and they threw the book at him. Lyle figured that this was better than getting shot by an angry dealer.

Over the next several days, as Lyle's mind cleared, and as my withdrawals were just beginning, Lyle and I became inseparable. Superficially, we couldn't have been more different, but it's astounding what we had in common. We were both medical professionals with failing marriages, who entered the same rehab at the same time, for addiction to the same molecule. We were in the same amount of trouble, with the same challenges and timelines. We were the same age and had the same attitude and sense of humor.

It was as if the same person had been born into two different lives, with divergent evolution for forty years, and then suddenly transported into the same habitat. We were on the same wavelength.

Lyle had a natural gift for lightening things up, charming himself out of trouble, and finding the humor in any situation. He could cheer anyone up, and often zeroed in on the new arrivals, who were limping along, to do just that. He would flirt with the overweight secretaries, who were bored and lonely at their jobs, just enough to leave them with a smile.

Lyle's ebullience and wit helped me from descending into gloom, especially when I was thinking about how far away I was from my kids and how fun it was to wrestle with them, read them picture books, or take them to the beach, which is what I would have been doing if I weren't locked up.

We were allowed to use telephones during the day, but they were all fixed to the same wall in the main lobby. This was to prevent private conversations, so that no one could set up a drug deal or a tryst. We heard each other's dirty laundry, which, in its way, made us all closer.

One week into my stay, I was on the receiving end of a withering diatribe from H. No "Are you feeling OK?" or "What's it like down there?" Her voice was literally booming across the open spaces, at a skull-shattering volume and pitch. "You fucking drug addict...you deserve everything that is happening to you...I'm going to serve you with [divorce] papers!"

Lyle approached me, grinning, and asked, "Don't that hurt your hearing? It hurts mine, way over in the lounge. You can hear her from Boston. Sounds like she really misses you."

Lyle's marriage, like mine, was "up shit's creek." He had met Sandra about four years earlier, when she was nineteen. At that time, she was a waitress at Hooters and, in a tight shirt and short shorts, was the "Hooters Girl" assigned to accompany Lyle and his friends during a drunken Hooters golf celebration. It was lust at first sight, and he determined to "put a ring on her finger before someone else did."

They did well at first but gradually, over several years, Sandra began sensing that Lyle was checking out. Oxycontin became more important to him than anything else, and he paid less and less attention to her. He was staying up all night, secretly snorting, and sleeping most of the time he wasn't working. He also had slowly drained their bank account to support his drug dealer. He smashed up their Beemer.

When Sandra came to visit Tannenberg, she was shocked to see that Lyle was spending what little was left of their money on "this

country club." She had envisioned a crude and punitive environment for his penance, as payback for his snorting up their life. To
this day, even though they are doing well, and now have a beautiful daughter, Sandra doesn't fully believe that Lyle was joking
when he mentioned the hot tub, the golf course, and the masseuse.

While at Greenpeace, just like at college, I was intermittently
afflicted with anxiety and depression. The stimulating adventures I
was participating in distracted me from these symptoms but didn't
make them disappear. I suspect the drugs did the same thing.

On summer evenings, when there weren't any Greenpeace
parties, and I didn't have any concrete plans, I took to wandering
the streets of the Mount Pleasant and Adams Morgan neighborhoods of Washington, DC, consumed with a restless loneliness.
Instead of being at home, content with a book or with my own
company, I'd walk and wander, feeling more alone with each
house party I'd pass, many of them spilling outside into the tem-
perate DC air. Sometimes I'd enter, but that made it worse, not
knowing anyone, feeling like an interloper, watching the others
dance and laugh.

These feelings were gaining in intensity, and I thought I best
resume seeing a psychiatrist. I was referred to a Harvard class-
mate of my dad's, Dr. Goldstein, an expert in Otto Rank, who
was one of Freud's disciples, and who championed the importance
of birth trauma. Having been traumatized by my own birth, or
at least shortly afterward when Martin got to go home and I was
stuck in an incubator, I thought he was a good choice.

Dr. Goldstein was also politically sympathetic; he was almost
kicked out of Harvard for refusing to sign a loyalty oath in the
1950s. He was good-natured when I teased him about Otto Rank
and how silly the idea of birth trauma is.

"Wasn't Anaïs Nin his patient?"
"Yes."
"Didn't he fuck her?"
"Well, yes, he did."

"I thought that was the *one thing* a psychiatrist isn't sup-
posed to do with a patient."
*"Well, um, er, that's technically true, but he was still a brilliant
psychiatrist."*
"Haven't Freud and his disciples gone by the wayside?"
"Many of their ideas are still valid."
"But birth trauma. You have to be kidding. No one even
remembers their birth."
*"There's reason to believe it's important. Let's focus on your
therapy now."*

Dr. Goldstein pointed out that, whenever presented with a
choice, I chose the more stressful option in order to make life feel
more interesting and meaningful, the whole Danny and the Art
thing. Not surprisingly, many of these choices were contributing
to my stress. Case in point: It would ultimately be less stressful to rejoin life's conveyor belt, go to medical school, and settle
down, rather than remain at Greenpeace with a low salary and an
unknown future.

Dr. Goldstein thought that my insomnia and depression were
partly biochemical and could be improved by medication. Prozac
was very new at the time, and relatively untested, so he chose an
old faithful, Valium, mother's little helper, to improve my mood
swings and quiet my anxiety.

Dr. Goldstein couldn't possibly have known at that point that
I was an addiction waiting to happen, even if the major mani-
festations of the addiction weren't to erupt for another decade.
If he could go back in time after viewing the wreckage, maybe
he would have chosen a less addictive drug. I don't blame him.
It was a good drug for me at the time, given my level of anxiety.

The problem is that it was too good a drug for me. Its chemical
structure had a too-good affinity with my particular brain cells.
It made me just a little bit too relaxed and happy.

When I initially arrived at Tannenberg, my bottle of Klonapin
was confiscated by Nurse Jasmin. In the Tannenberg jurisdiction,

Klonapin was as invalid as heroin, pot, or methamphetamine, even if presented with a valid prescription.

"You are a drug addict, and you can never take any of these medications again. No Klonapin and no Valium. No painkillers. No abusable medicines. We will help you through this transition."

"What if I break my leg?"

"Don't break your leg."

This seemed dogmatic to me, and with this confiscation, I realized that their dogma was about to affect my karma. "It's gonna get ya, yeah, yeah, yeah."

The prospect of going cold turkey off the Klonapin terrified me. In this case, knowledge was not power, but learned helplessness. I knew the withdrawal syndrome from Klonapin can last up to eighteen months, with a risk of seizures. I had no choice but to follow instructions and cross my fingers that they didn't botch this up. Doctors are *not* good at being patients, and I had a hard time putting my trust in the staff. Rehab facilities don't necessarily attract the cutting edge of Western medicine.

I had been prescribed either Klonapin or Valium for my entire adult life. I used it every night. If I didn't take it, I didn't sleep at all. Period. Ironically, these are the drugs that got me tagged on my drug screen and landed me in rehab, not the opiates, which had hijacked my life.

The Valium was originally started by Dr. Goldstein when I was twenty-three, fifteen years earlier, and had been changed to its cousin Klonapin by my third psychiatrist. The dosage had been gradually creeping up over the years. I encouraged this process as much as possible. I said, "I'm so anxious, I can't sleep, I think I need just one more milligram each night." My dose went from two to three to four to five milligrams, which is a huge dose.

I had been supplementing the Klonapin prescription with whatever I could get my hands on. They were going to detox me from five milligrams, but I was really taking more like eight to ten. I didn't want to implicate myself by telling them this. I just steeled myself for a bumpy and unpleasant ride.

To stop body and mind from getting too hyperactive off the Klonapin, and to prevent seizures, I was put on hefty doses of three different tranquilizers: phenobarbital (a barbiturate that makes everything dreamlike), Neurontin (which slows down nerve impulses and makes even simple thoughts take longer than they should), and Seroquel (an antipsychotic medication ordinarily given to schizophrenics and manic-depressives to dampen their abnormal brain activity and make them calmer).

The first time I took this combination of medications, I fell asleep midsentence during a conversation with Lyle, slumped in my chair. The next morning, he asked, "Where'd you go? All of a sudden you went zombie on me, rolled your eyes, and were gone."

The Seroquel alone made me feel like I had just arrived from outer space. This combination of medications initially made me feel as lively as a potted plant. I came to sympathize with all of the frogs I pithed in high school biology lab. My thoughts were fragmented. It didn't feel like progress to be placed on all of these drugs in the service of getting me off all of those other drugs. What hypocrites! Hardest was that I had no say in the matter.

This lethargy didn't last long. The first withdrawal symptom started on my fourth day, as my body continued to degrade the Klonapin that was stored in my fat. I noticed a gradually escalating feeling of restlessness, as if I had drunk first four or five, then a dozen shots of espresso. Feet tapping, hands tapping, legs shaking, I was radiating restless energy. It was hard to find a comfortable position. I was uncomfortable in my skin.

Over the next few days, still during my first week there, as my energy thermostat kept readjusting upward, I started having racing thoughts and drenching sweats. I couldn't think clearly, and everyone around me seemed to be moving in slow motion. I was in a different time zone, like the *Star Trek* episode where some of the crew were sped up and were perceived by the others only as a buzzing sound.

Southerners speak slowly, which is why, unfairly, they have a reputation for being dumb. This slowness of speech can be frustrating under normal circumstances to a quick-witted and impatient Yankee. But in my situation, with them speaking at two miles per hour and my brain listening at one thousand, it was getting ridiculous. The coal miners were the worst offenders: "My... friend...'n... I... were... in... the... truck... with... the... dog...'nd... the... wife... at... home... goin'... after... work... down... to... see..." Just finish your goddamn sentence, already! I'll finish it for you. Hurry the fuck up, before I slit my throat!

With fifteen years of Klonapin and Valium wearing off, few would dispute the fact that I was becoming manic. My words spilled out faster and faster, and I'd be seen zooming down the hallway, unshaven, unkempt, and talking a mile a minute.

When I told my new friend Helen, a playful and intelligent nurse practitioner (who, after five years sober, stole some fentanyl from the ER where she worked, and overdosed in a locked closet), that I had a twin brother, she replied in a clinical, patronizing voice, "*Sure* you do," convinced that I was delusional and that I was talking about an imaginary friend. One of the other guests, Zeke, complained that he "cain't understand a damn thing [he is saying]" and that he hoped "all Yankees ain't *nuts*."

The feeling was somewhat mutual. Zeke was a tall, wiry, edentulous, God-fearing, but affectionate coal miner from Kentucky, with messy long hair, a dense southern accent, and a nasty Oxycontin habit. Zeke was the most cadaverous-looking person I'd met. He reminded me of my cadaver from anatomy class, with its cold, unreal flesh. Maybe all of the cigarettes and coal dust helped preserve him.

At home in West Virginia, while ascending from the mines, Zeke routinely got blasted with his recovery sponsor. With his sponsor! Why bother going through the motions? Why not just admit and accept that you are on drugs?

This was Zeke's fourth attempt at rehab. Any interaction between Zeke and me was dependent on Lyle serving as a translator between southern coal-miner language, slurred by his lack of teeth, and, from his perspective, my rapid-paced, multisyllabic, "nuts" Yankee speech.

Zeke was a "professional patient," someone so experienced with rehab programs that he knew by rote exactly what to say and how to act. His passionate, meandering, quasi-coherent locutions were works of art. Without warning, his eyes would close, his brows would furrow in concentration, and his body would evince a barely perceptible tremor; sounding like a fully possessed evangelist speaking in tongues, Zeke would fall prostrate: "All ya have ta do is accept God's love and get down on yer knees to find freed'm from drugs... *On yer knees, y'all!*" He always looked surprised and disappointed that none of us ever joined him on the ground.

The physicians at Tannenberg who managed my withdrawal were skilled and competent. I was uncomfortable, but they helped me survive the transition away from the ungodly amount of sedatives I was taking. The nurse practitioner Patricia, on the other hand, was somewhat of a hazard and an obstacle.

I first met Patricia a week into my rehab sojourn. She was blond, slim and athletic, primly dressed, about five feet five, and I was just starting to launch into a sexual fantasy about her when I heard her metallic, drill-sergeant voice, and my newborn reverie came flopping down. "Peter, now that you are stable, I'm in charge of your meds." Oh, crap.

Many nurse practitioners resent doctors, a cumulative response to decades of being on the receiving end of doctor arrogance and abuse. In rehab, they have absolute power over you.

After speaking with me for a few minutes, Patricia said, "You look jumpy," and put in an order to increase the dose of both my phenobarbital and my Seroquel. I protested, because, just that morning, Dr. Garber had already made this same change. Patricia instantly became enraged and barked, "Don't you dare question my orders, or I'll report you for noncompliance and you'll never get back to the practice of medicine."

That night, when the nurses provided my plastic cup containing my nightly pills, they insisted that I swallow the pills in front of them so that they could witness that I was complying with orders. Patricia had tipped them off, and they hate it when know-it-all doctors second-guess them.

I counted the pills: three reds, six small pinks, and three whites. As I feared, it was not double but *triple* the doses of all of the medications—enough to put Godzilla to sleep in the middle of snacking on Tokyo.

I asked them to call Patricia, then Dr. Garber, which they refused to do. The option of not taking these pills just wasn't on the menu of my available responses. At rehab, you can't petition for conscientious objector status or opt out of medical require- ments you don't agree with. It's also not like the movies, where the clever protagonist secrets the pills under his or her tongue and spits them out later. This is almost impossible to do in real life, especially with trained and suspicious nurses watching you.

After swallowing the pills, I called my twin to tell him what happened, just in case, so he could sue them and put Annie and Milo through college if I didn't wake up. Twenty minutes later, according to Lyle, I pulled another zombie, upright in a chair, midsentence, and then slept for twelve hours. "You were goin' on with your normal nonsense, then the next moment you were gone. I couldn't wake you up."

When she found out the next day, Patricia first said "Oops," then "I'm so sorry." It's hard not to forgive a sincere apology, though later she furiously backpedaled to avoid looking incom- petent in front of the doctors, and blamed me for not accurately describing my symptoms.

At the noon lecture, I was overwhelmingly groggy from this overdose. The day nurses accused me of experiencing a "change in mental status." No shit—you poisoned me last night. Ignoring my explanation, and suspecting that I had relapsed, they ordered an extra drug screen and sent me directly to the lab. They watched me carefully as I peed into the proverbial cup.

After this test, the lab technician offered me some alcohol- based disinfectant to clean my hands, because the sink wasn't working. As I was walking back toward the lecture room, a dif- ferent nurse, farther down the hallway, smelled the disinfectant and accused me of having alcohol on my breath. Ignoring my lat- est explanation, she ordered me to go back, again, to the lab for a Breathalyzer test. By this point, I was running on fumes, and feared that I was caught in an infinite regress between different groups of nurses, strategically placed to avoid my getting any rest.

Over the next few days, I started to adjust myself to the "academic" portions of my rehab program. It was through an alchemy of group therapy, workshops, and recovery meetings that we were supposed to cross the threshold from druggie to recovered.

A central part of our recovery diet was group therapy, which we would participate in daily for the final ten weeks of rehab. I stumbled into my first therapy group utterly brain-dead from the medicines they were giving me, and increasingly manic from my withdrawal from the Klonapin. Classic mania involves hyperreligiosity, hypersexuality, and grandiosity of thought. I was mostly just hyper, with thought after thought spilling out of my mouth, ideas that might not be connected to the conversation or to what I had just said. I knew this was happening but had lost my ability to edit, filter, and, mostly, to slow down.

My image of a therapy group was of cooperative, articulate peers calmly deconstructing their pasts to figure out where their addictions had taken hold. This group would be led by a gentle counselor who resembled in comportment the sympathetic, Harvard-trained therapists I'd had in the past.

I walked into a small room with six seats in a circle, all facing a desk, like a throne, where Nate, my counselor, was sitting. When I eyeballed Nate, I temporarily lost faith. Nate was a huge, imposing man, ex-military, ex-biker, potbellied, graying, bearded, and balding. He was dressed in clothing that had transitioned over the years from biker chic to rags. He sported an expression somewhere between sarcastic and homicidal.

Nate looked at me suspiciously and demanded, "Who are you?" "I'm Peter Grinspoon." I thought about adding "sir" but I knew that would piss him off. "Peter, what are you doing here?" I told him that I was in rehab, and that he was my therapist. He paused for a moment, and tried to clarify.

"No, how did you get here?"

"I drove down from Boston, sir."

On hearing this, Nate visibly lost patience. "No, you *idiot*, why are you here in rehab?" They were teaching us that honesty was the best policy. "My lawyer told me that I had to be here looking like I was getting better, if I wanted to practice medicine again." Nate responded: "Listen, I'm not supposed to injure you, so just tell us what you did to end up in rehab. I don't give a fuck about when you were potty-trained, 'less it was done at gunpoint."

I then gave a bewildering (even to me), jumpy, free-associational speech, which touched upon the traumas of my childhood in a psychiatric family, including the death of my brother Danny, a summary of all of my different therapists in the past, what they thought my problems were, what I thought were their limitations as therapists, why marijuana isn't really a drug that contributes to addiction, and how I am absolutely convinced that religion is the opiate of the masses. I concluded by saying, "It doesn't make sense to trade one drug for another."

Nate scratched his head and said, "You seem to be in the right place, though you're gonna intellect'lyze yerself, and the rest of us, to death. You know lots in yer head, but you don't know shit in your heart. They don't seem to be connected."

To break the glacier-level ice, he said, "What you need ta know 'bout North Carolina is that it ain't Massachusetts. People here think that the show *Hee Haw* is a documentary." Laughter eased the tension. He proceeded to introduce me to my therapy group, which included, in addition to Lyle, Felix, Tony, Brett, and Adam, a diverse and motley crew.

Felix had been a petty officer in the navy. He had curly brown hair and a repressed, military demeanor, like a dog that has been beaten one too many times. He thought that anyone opposed to the first Gulf War, or any military action by our government, was a "bed wetter." He was completely immune to logic or history.

Felix had absolutely no self-confidence and was a veritable volcano of pent-up anger and resentment. Without friends or family, utterly alone, he would spend every weekend with a case of beer in different hotel rooms, drinking by himself and watching TV until he managed to drink enough to fall asleep.

Felix's job was guarding prisoners in a state penitentiary. One day, without warning, he snapped, and became irrational and threatening with them, which triggered an evaluation that concluded in a diagnosis of severe alcoholism and a free ticket to rehab. Our tax dollars at work. The Tea Party's paranoid fantasy had come true. (Actually, their paranoid fantasy would probably be paying for Big Bird at rehab...) His career and pension were on the line, so he had external motivation to recover.

Tony was pleasant, handsome, dark-featured, Italian, a plumber by vocation who worked in his family's business and would do absolutely anything to get high. His family sent him to rehab as he increasingly screwed up on the job, and everywhere else. He once tried snorting Prozac to get high, thinking that if it can cause happiness in pill form, snorting would be even better. Sorry, Tony, Prozac uses a different set of receptors than Oxycontin or cocaine, and can't get you high.

Adam, an ER doc, was kind and intelligent, with all of the external trappings of his sexual orientation. Midmarriage, with two kids, in his thirties, he realized that he was gay and, feeling trapped, started having secret affairs and became increasingly involved with the gay methamphetamine sex scene.

After an initially brutal divorce, Adam's ex-wife came to accept that his defection from their marriage was hardwired into his nature, and not a deliberate rejection. They were able to mend their relationship and coparent together harmoniously. But the addiction to methamphetamine spiraled out of control, which is always what happens with this evil drug.

Adam's final binge landed him in the same emergency department where he worked. He was hallucinating that everyone's hair was purple. Go directly to rehab. Do not pass Go.

My final group member, besides Lyle, was Brett, another ER doc. Brett was a Hispanic American, very tall, with a mustache, black hair, a jocular demeanor, and the insincere, slightly predatory personality that is stereotypically associated with used-car salesmen. He had an earsplitting, barking laugh, sounding like a herd of seals getting simultaneously electrocuted. Once, when I was sitting in close proximity to him, his laugh caused my right ear to buzz and become deaf for several minutes.

Brett's immediate addiction was to alcohol, but I believe a much more serious problem was that he, at heart, was a phony and a liar. He was vastly more of a bullshitter than me and the other addicts. He was operating on a different plane of dishonesty.

Brett would proudly boast that when trying to pick up Caucasian women in bars, he'd lay on the Hispanic accent and pretend to be a rich Mexican aristocrat. He'd do the opposite with Hispanic women.

During the "family weekend," he was visited by his, according to him, "white trash" girlfriend. She was a single mom of a two-year-old. She was clinging to him for dear life, clinging to him as tightly as her Daisy Dukes clung to her butt. She was hoping to one day become a doctor's wife and have security for her kid. Behind her back, Brett stated that he was using her, temporarily, while he was in rehab, that he didn't care about her at all, and that he was intending to dump her the moment he got out. We were all up in arms about this, but there wasn't anything we could do.

As I got to know other doctors in recovery, all of whom had been through so much suffering, I reflected back to one of my first patient visits in my new job out of residency. This patient was a young man, tall, scruffy, dressed in the blue surgical scrubs of an anesthesiology resident. Looking tired and washed out, ashamed but somehow defiant, he came in with paperwork to be filled out. The paperwork was from an organization called Society to Help Physicians, which I hadn't heard of yet.

This patient requested that I, through signing, attest that I was his primary care doctor and that I was aware of the fact that he was in a monitoring contract with Society to Help Physicians as part of his recovery from drug abuse.

He was in the process of restarting his contract because of a relapse. He said, "I didn't know that cough syrup had codeine in it." Give me a break! Like an anesthesiologist wouldn't know that. Can't you come up with anything better?

What still amazes me is how I approached him not with compassion and empathy, or an attempt to understand him, or how I could help him, but with supercilious scorn and condescension. Is that how my doctors looked at me when I crashed and burned?

My attitude to this doctor was phenomenally hypocritical, because by that time I was:

- Writing prescriptions for Percocet in the name of my medical assistant and having her fill them and give me the pills.
- Pilfering freely from our supply closet and having the pharmaceutical companies send me samples of Tramadol (a painkiller), Provigil, and Meridia (stimulants for weight loss).
- Snooping through the other doctors' offices in the building, looking for medication samples, searching their desks for bottles of pills.
- Returning to my office at night and inhaling hits off the tank of nitrous oxide in the neighboring doctor's office.
- Calling in prescriptions to CVS in H.'s name and picking them up on my way home from work, posing as her dutiful husband. (She figured this out and instructed CVS not to let me pick up any of her prescriptions, and threatened to go to the medical board, and then the police, if I did it again.)

I wondered if all addicted healthcare professionals faced similarly crappy attitudes as they sought help.

Nate started off the group by saying, "You all feel bad right now, like failures. When you think about it, you aren't really a failure 'til you're six feet in the ground and they are shoveling dirt on your face. If you're still breathing, you still have time to pull this together."

He had us report on how we were feeling physically, mentally, emotionally, and spiritually. I said, "Physically, I feel like crap. Mentally, I can't think because of the drugs you're giving me.

Emotionally, I'm bored and angry. And spiritually, I'm an atheist who doesn't fall for any of this religious crap." I was hoping to get a rise out of him, but he chuckled and moved on.

Nate was able to lead this therapy group by example because he was at heart one of us. In his pre-therapist past, he had rerouted his windshield wiper fluid dispenser to drain into the cab of his car, and then filled it up with vodka instead of wiper fluid. Being from the South, where it is socially acceptable to work on a car all day, he'd drink with abandon while his wife blithely thought he was pursuing a constructive hobby. It wasn't long until he was sipping vodka from the windshield wiper dispenser while driving, and was arrested for a repeat DUI.

In jail, Nate had a spiritual conversion, which led to his recovery. Now, as a counselor, he was living proof of the ancient adage "You can't bullshit a bullshitter." Oh, did I try, with the full force of my intellect. For the first time, someone could see right through me.

Nate thought I was a snob who used big words deliberately to bamboozle and intimidate. I informed him that his conceptual paradigm was maladroitly expostulated and intellectually vacant. He looked like he was going to club me senseless.

Nate hated my tendency to "overintellectualize" and thought it was my biggest obstacle in recovery. "For you, the longest distance is 'tween yer heart and yer brain. You need a sponsor with a third-grade education, to stop you from thinking so much, who can tell you to shut your mouth when you start spewing these big words."

Great: My sponsor can coach me on recovery and I can teach him how to read. We could start with *Go, Dog. Go!* I could borrow this from my daughter, Annie, who was five. Now, why would Nate think I'm a snob?

Nate said that to recover, I had to believe either in myself or in God. When he found out I was a diehard atheist, he let fly: "What's the definition of a dead atheist? All dressed up, nowhere to go." He said I reminded him of Mister Rogers. Once, I was really upset with him for dumping on me in group, and I starting yelling at him. He started sobbing with laughter. "It's just too funny being yelled at by Mister Rogers. It's a *beautiful* day in the neighborhood, Grinspoon."

Nate hammered away at my identity as a doctor, and helped me to rediscover who I was without the protective, distorting shield of a medical degree and before my addiction had corroded my character. He said my job is "what you do, not who you are."

I had bumped into this idea years before, when visiting my twin brother on a Native American reservation in New Mexico, where he worked as an attorney. Trying to make small talk at a party on the "res," I offended several people by asking them what they did for a living. Few of them had jobs. One of them informed me, gravely, "You don't ask that here."

Many of my discussions with Nate centered around when my addiction started. Was it when Dr. Goldstein first prescribed Valium for my anxiety when I worked for Greenpeace? Or was it later, in medical school, when I stumbled upon Vicodin? Or was I showing addictive behavior at Swarthmore with excessive caffeine, tobacco, Benadryl, and with my experimentation with mushrooms, acid, and Ecstasy? Perhaps I just hadn't collided with my drug of choice yet.

Or did my addiction begin even earlier? To this date, I'm skeptical about whether my marijuana use in junior high school and high school contributed to my later addiction to opiates. I seemed to do fine with occasional marijuana use, in school and socially, and I didn't struggle with addiction until I was introduced to prescription drugs several decades later. At the time, marijuana seemed to promote togetherness and creativity with my friends, and didn't impact my schoolwork, except perhaps to improve the quality of my writing.

Some addiction "experts" tout research that purports to show that marijuana use in adolescence is associated with substance abuse later on, which, if true, would evidence that cannabis did pave the way for my later addiction. But these data seem thin at best (though, to be safe, no one advocates that adolescents use cannabis). Addiction "experts" are so ideologically and politically opposed to cannabis that it's hard to distinguish real information from propaganda. They have thoroughly brainwashed themselves on this issue, and somehow seem to know less about the pros and cons of marijuana usage than your average cannabis-consuming adult layperson.

One could make an argument that, behaviorally, becoming an inveterate pothead so early in life might have dismantled various barriers against breaking the law, which made it easier to disregard the law as a doctor, when my addiction started gaining momentum. Also, at an early age, I picked up the habit of using substances to escape reality and to feel better. This habit was ingrained too early, and too deeply, to change.

I can imagine that possibly, the stage was being set, with one prop being the teenage marijuana and another being the Ecstasy in college. The Valium was best supporting actor. The star of the show wasn't to come onstage until medical school.

Nate gave me a few days to "learn the ropes" at Tannenberg, which largely meant figuring out with Lyle how to avoid getting into trouble, so we wouldn't get restricted or reported. With good behavior, there was a gradual increase in personal freedom, freedom I had enjoyed right until admission to Tannenberg. It was like getting to wear a Pull-Up if you can keep your diaper clean for several days in a row.

Once I was over the acute throes of detox and deemed medically stable, and the staff felt my behavior was halfway responsible, I would be eligible to graduate to "stage 2," living in the off-campus apartments with the guys.

Almost everyone at rehab smokes cigarettes, even diehard asthmatics who struggle with each breath to capture enough oxygen to remain conscious. By far the most reliable outcome of rehab is an addiction to nicotine. It took me a full five minutes to develop a half-a-pack-per-day nicotine habit. All of the doctors and nurses smoked. We smoked as a consolation, to fill the time, and to satisfy addiction-hungry neurons that weren't getting what they really wanted. Everyone said I looked ridiculous with a cigarette in my mouth. Nate said I looked like Mister Rogers with a cigarette, and cracked a smile every time he walked by.

A typical day at Tannenberg began with Lyle over our morning cigarettes and coffee. Lyle would greet me:

"Good mornin', Grinspoon, you clean and sober yet?"
"More sober every second that passes. What about you?"
"I'm still thinking about Hooters last night."
"Lyle, you've got to focus."
"I am focusing...on that blonde in Hooters last night."
"Lyle, each one of her body parts was fake. She was held
   together with Elmer's glue."
"And it's a great thing too."

Lyle and I stuck together to avoid breaking the "no spending time alone" rule. The only exception to this rule was when you had to go to the bathroom. At least number two didn't have to be supervised by the nurses, like number one was during the drug tests.

We smoked and socialized in "the garden," a walled-off weed patch that hosted a meager collection of plastic chairs, worn tables, and unkempt plants. One of the other patients, a gardener by trade, started weeding the garden and picking up trash, until he was forced to stop by the nurses because this violated the "do not practice your vocation while in rehab" rule. Give me a break!

The visibility in this garden area ranged from about three to eight feet, depending on local weather conditions, because it was perpetually enveloped in clouds of cigarette smoke. It was easier to hear the other people than to see them. It took several days to associate faces with voices.

After the cigarette break, we'd rush to get some coffee before they switched it over to decaf, part of the "no caffeine after 8:00 a.m. because you need to learn to live without stimulants and other mind-altering chemicals" rule. This forced us to chug coffee and hide cups of it in our room for later. After coffee, we'd mill around for them to announce the daily list of who gets a drug test.

The next part of the morning would be consumed by a "lecture," usually some warmed-over AA platitudes, repeated again and again in lecture format. I would smuggle a novel into the lectures and sit in back.

One frequent lecture was on "Letting go and letting God." I still don't understand what that meant. Letting God do what? Letting God hold on to whatever you were letting go of? Did it mean that you let God have a turn, like with a new toy? Or letting God catch something before it fell and hit the ground, after you let go, like a trust fall? Everyone else was nodding enthusiastically, so I just let it go (and let God). Maybe this was what religion was all about, and it was very significant and meaningful, but invisible to me.

Almost all of the staff members at Tannenberg, from doctors and nurses down to support staff, were themselves in recovery. The cook, a tough, garrulous, middle-aged black woman named Bella, barked out encouragements such as "One day at a time" or "Progress not perfection" from the kitchen while preparing our meals.

This pervasive recovery ethos was a two-edged sword. On the one hand, it was encouraging to see these same staff members at the local AA meetings, attending voluntarily, as peers. I didn't feel judged or looked down upon at all during my entire three-month stay, and I felt a strong bond that I otherwise wouldn't have felt. On the other hand, at times it felt like a cult. It made for a lot of repetition during the piss-poor lectures, structure without content, preaching to the converted.

After the lecture, the guys bundled into their trucks and went to the local community center and pumped iron. We did this at a different time of day from the women, to avoid breaking the "only interact with the opposite gender with strict supervision" rule. This restriction felt like it was being beamed to us from Victorian England. Over time, I came to understand that relationships formed in rehab tend to fail, and destroy families along the way.

Away from your family, rehab is a hellishly lonely place, but hooking up with another homesick addict in early recovery, with an equally shattered life, can vastly compound a person's problems. When you are alone and sex-starved, you can idealize the attractive people around you, and your spouse can seem very far away, and frumpy, part of a different world.

Doris, a pretty southern-belle oncology nurse, was in rehab for her unfortunate habit of stealing Demerol from patients and injecting it into the skin on her thighs, which heavily scarred an otherwise flawless beauty. She was constantly applying hand cream so she wouldn't reek of cigarettes.

Doris learned about rehab love the hard way, after a two-week clandestine romance with a strikingly handsome but immature and brainless coal miner named Willis. She ended up pregnant just as it was time to graduate from Tannenberg and confront the shambles of her previous life. It was against her religion and culture to terminate this pregnancy, and Willis promptly ditched her when his own rehab term was up. She went back to live with her parents.

The "no fraternizing with the opposite gender" rule was strictly enforced, and easy to innocently break because it was so counterintuitive. Once, a few of us happened to enter Starbucks when our female counterparts were there. We sat at a table outside and drank our coffees together, like any normal adults would do. Later that night, we were separately interrogated. I was repeatedly asked, "*Who* orchestrated the rendezvous at Starbucks?" as if we were some terrorist cell plotting an imminent attack on critical infrastructure.

After exercise, we went to our daily Narcotics Anonymous or Alcoholics Anonymous meeting, held in the basements of Baptist and other churches, which, except for their basements, were incredibly opulent, with sparkling windows, expensive cars in the parking lot, impeccable landscaping, and enormous crosses out front, boldly and defiantly proclaiming the fervency of their devotion.

The basements, where the addicts and drunks were hidden, had dirty floors, stained ceilings, glaring fluorescent lights, and uncomfortable plastic chairs. It was where they had located the day care, so toys were scattered all around. They served instant coffee in Styrofoam cups with artificial creamer, which unfailingly burned through my stomach. Down-and-out alcoholics would mumble the same old lines from the AA playbook, one day at a time, year after year, trying to stay off the sauce.

We were required by Tannenberg to participate, so I would say, "My name is Peter and I am a drug addict" and then give lip service to the topic at hand, be it "Gratitude" or "Knowing Yourself" or "Living a Sober Life." At the time, I couldn't care less. I was bored and angry.

The spring was spectacular at Tannenberg, with a bright green, lush, sickly sweet–smelling jungle of vegetation sprouting everywhere, before the deathly hot heat of summer began. With the sun peeking through the grime of the basement windows, hinting at what was going on outside, my mind would start to wander, and it was all but impossible for me to sit through the meetings. The freshness of these mornings was somewhat diminished by the smell of tobacco smoke on everyone's clothing. (North Carolina is tobacco country, so you are encouraged, from birth, to chew, spit, and snuff tobacco.)

It was especially difficult given how slowly everyone in the South speaks, which made a ninety-minute meeting seem more like four hours. The nature of these meetings is fundamentally based on repetition, which was torture to my analytical, knowledge-hungry mind. If it were possible to die of boredom, I would have perished long ago in one of those North Carolina basements.

Many of the meetings were dominated by Jeb, a local good ol' boy who looked like Charlie Daniels or some guy from ZZ Top with his long, gray beard, wild eyes, and homespun expressions. Daily, he would lament that being an alcoholic was "'bout as sad as bein' a one-legg'd man in a butt-kickin' contest."

Jeb's other favorite saying, uttered when people used the meetings as a forum to complain about their lives, was "Alcoholics Anonymous ain't Self-Help Anonymous, so stop yer goddamn bellyaching." Jeb's characteristic gesticulations, arms raised with all fingers wiggling, remain a secret code for all who have experienced Jeb the world over. I would see this code flashed many years later at recovery meetings at the Society to Help Physicians back in Boston, by sober doctors.

Unlike meetings up in Boston, to my utter shock and horror these meetings closed with everyone standing up, holding hands, looking devout, and reciting not the Serenity Prayer, but an actual prayer, the Lord's Prayer, in unison, which goes, for those of you, like me, who had never heard it before:

> *Our Father, which art in heaven,*
> *Hallowed be thy Name.*
> *Thy Kingdom come.*
> *Thy will be done in earth,*
> *As it is in heaven.*
> *Give us this day our daily bread.*
> *And forgive us our trespasses,*
> *As we forgive those who trespass against us.*
> *And lead us not into temptation,*
> *But deliver us from evil.*
> *For thine is the kingdom,*
> *The power, and the glory,*
> *For ever and ever.*
> *Amen.*

I felt like screaming, "I'm Jewish! I'm an atheist. This is bullshit." These group prayer sessions reinforced all of my most paranoid fantasies of rehab being a Christian indoctrination, though I remembered it being even worse at Talbott in Atlanta, which was farther south. Down there, I felt like we had Mass and got baptized each morning.

I refused to participate, couldn't participate, and would discreetly sneak out before this part of the meetings. Nate, hearing this, made me read the chapter in the AA Bible "On Atheism," which I doubt he had actually read, because it essentially argued, by repetition, that atheists were lost souls who just hadn't found God yet. Not helpful.

After the AA meeting, we could drive back to the Tannenberg main campus to see what was next on that day's agenda, or we could find pay phones, a vanishing species, to call in to the mother ship.

Just after lunch was group with Nate, and after that, if it was a Wednesday, we would attend the men's support group. This was held in the off-campus apartments, which looked and smelled like a fraternity, except instead of beer there was soda.

Behind closed doors, over chips and pretzels, many of the guys, once they exhausted the usual topics of which of the female patients they wanted to fuck, or wouldn't ever fuck, or would fuck if they were drunk, or for money, or out of mercy, would start blaming "the niggers" for the world's problems. I was in the cultural minority and was unsure whether to speak up. I didn't want to be an outcast for the ten weeks that remained, and I was not sanguine about changing a master/slave mentality that had been ingrained for hundreds of years. There were no African Americans in this rehab, at least when I was there.

Lyle seemed torn between his loyalty to me and to the rest of the world he lived in. He said to the guys, "We're starting to get them [niggers] over in my part of the state," as if he was talking about some plague. Later, looking guilty, he said to me, "People down here aren't so open-minded as where you're from." True dat.

Phil was a pharmacist from North Carolina who was jovial and suave, with an athletic build and classic good looks, but was plainly dumb. He had been tagged for a prescription violation while feeding his habit, caught with his hand in the cookie jar. (I wonder how pharmacists ever learn to resist this type of temptation. They are surrounded by pills all day.) Evidently bored with "the niggers," Phil started blaming "the Jews" for the financial problems he was having, not that getting fired from his job and spending all of his money on drugs could have had anything to do with it. He was completely oblivious to the fact that I was Jewish. Afterward, flushed with embarrassment, he apologized to me, though by that time I had already decided he was a Nazi and wouldn't have anything to do with him.

On Monday nights we would have a "Caduceus" meeting, restricted to doctors and nurses, about thirty of us sitting in a large circle under the vaulted ceiling and grand windows of the main meeting room. In this meeting, we would discuss our feelings as failed professionals and share different strategies for managing our *persona non grata* status at the medical and nursing boards. I looked forward to these meetings, because misery loves company and solidarity. Sometimes we were joined by former Tannenberg inmates who were now back in practice, in order to inspire us with the hope that there was light at the end of the tunnel. One of them relapsed during my stay, and became a patient again.

Linda, a senior Tannenberg nurse who ran these meetings, a tall, stately woman of sixty, with a compassionate demeanor and just enough of an attitude for me to see that she must have been a major handful as a teen drug addict, advised, "It's important to distinguish between honesty and the truth. Honesty is when you tell them you made a mistake, you regret your actions, and you are committed to doing better in the future. The truth is when you tell them every little detail, and they use it to stop you from ever working again."

We would end our days sitting around the television in the common room, an open room cluttered with newspapers, recovery literature, and junk food. Some nights Al, an overweight podiatrist with an escalating alcohol problem, would strum his guitar, adding a mournful atmosphere. Several of the men would be arguing about sports, their arguments based on increasingly voluble repetition of the same few facts. Discreet flirting would be going on, with patients holding hands under the blankets on the sofa.

Lyle and I would wax philosophical. I opined, "I don't know why extremely fat women wear thongs to physical exams. It's gross. All their flesh is bulging out around the thong. I don't wear ballbuster underwear when I go to see my doctor, with my paunch hanging out. Why can't they wear regular underwear?"

"You ever consider, Grinspoon, maybe it wasn't a thong when they bought it, and they grew fatter, so it seems like a thong, but it ain't, and they are too cheap to buy new underwear, so it's the only underwear they own. Your 'posed to be liberal from Massachusetts. Have a heart."

As my Seroquel was kicking in, and as my thoughts started to slow and the world started to go blurry and fuzzy for the evening, I would feel a sense of harmony with the others. For a few minutes, as I was falling into sleep, thinking of my brothers, my parents, my cousins, my in-laws, who loved me and were rooting for me, listening to Lyle drone on, it seemed that, despite the shambles of my life that was awaiting me back in Boston, things were going to be OK.

Homing in on the specific and unique issues of physicians and addiction, as well as the pitfalls that awaited us in recovery, one of my first assignments from Nate was to discuss my time in medical school, including the ways in which this may have contributed to my addiction.

On the last day of anatomy class in medical school, after our final exam, we cleaned up the anatomy lab and disposed of the cadavers that we had so carefully cut apart over the previous nine months.

Unwisely, I smoked some strong marijuana before the cadaver cleanup. With my enhanced perceptions, I saw my classmates as a blur of frenetic activity, colorful ants scurrying robotically from task to task. They seemed soulless. We dumped the carcasses into plain wooden caskets, along with any spare, unattached body parts. It was like cleaning up after Thanksgiving. They had a service in the chapel for these corpses, as if religion was going to help them now they had been hacked to pieces by amateur medical students. Krazy Glue would have been more helpful.

The stresses of medical school were synergistic: academic pressure, poor nutrition, lack of sleep and exercise, lack of perspective, and the constant pressure of being evaluated. Some of the mentoring doctors threw tantrums, yelled, and humiliated medical students. The demands of medical school escalated during the third year, when our clinical rotations began. During certain stretches, I spent far more time in the hospital than out of it.

The surgical team I was assigned to once spent several hours trying to warm up a six-year-old boy who had fallen through the ice on a pond near his home. This involved flushing warm liquids into every body cavity we could, even putting him on a heart-lung bypass machine to speed the warming of his blood.

I was on my hands and knees under the surgical table with several other classmates, soaked, my back and knees throbbing, manually flushing warm water into syringes attached to tubes that ran into this small boy's body. To release their stress, the surgeons were viciously bellowing at us to work faster, as if we weren't working as quickly as we could in our horror and our panic.

This boy's temperature was eighty degrees when he came in, and we elevated it into the midnineties, but his heart never restarted. When it was "called," a sense of gloom settled on the operating room, along with the discarded vials, empty syringes, and bloodstained gauze that littered the floor. One of the nurses was weeping.

I volunteered to help take the body to where the family was waiting, after they had cleaned it up. I was so exhausted, sore, and numb, I had lost track of the big picture of what was going on, and was treating what I was about to do as yet one more task to complete for brownie points during this endless night.

I was utterly unprepared for the explosion of visceral wailing and keening that greeted us as the parents and siblings of the deceased made first contact with the body of what, a few hours earlier, must have been a happy, active boy asking permission to go out to play. Feeling vaguely guilty, I couldn't wait to leave the room.

Against this backdrop, with stress and exhaustion in all realms of life, it is easy to drift into a relationship with someone else who is desperately lonely. Medical school relationships do not tend to be the healthiest of relationships.

Tami was Japanese and seemed exotic, intelligent, and friendly. We spent countless hours studying together. When I visited Tami's family in southern Massachusetts, it was under the guise of "a friend," because it was taboo for her to date anyone Caucasian.

For the entire duration of my two-day visit, Tami's dad, a physician, sat in stony, brooding silence, while her mom, brother, and grandparents giggled at me whenever I spoke or moved. They gave me a traditional bean-paste candy, which, after a heroic effort to get it down, I gagged on and almost spit up. It tasted like beets, which reminded me of being at Chernobyl, and I burped up this taste for days.

At the dinner table, or sitting around the living room, there was absolutely no conversation, just an uncomfortable accusatory silence. Tami and her father weren't capable of talking to each other, but he invited us to his medical office in order to "shadow" him while he saw patients. This quickly became awkward when it was time for one of his patients' prostate exam.

After clinic, we visited a room, more like a shrine, under the main office, where Tami's dad stored all the samples of medicine from the pharmaceutical companies. He liked the idea of getting things for free, and this emporium of prescription medications went far beyond what I have seen in any hospital or other offices. Antibiotics, blood pressure medications, painkillers, allergy medicines; they had it all.

Tami had been complaining about a sore throat, so, upon our leaving, her mom and dad packed her a bag full to the brim with prescription medications. This was the main way that these silent parents communicated care and affection to their children.

After we returned home, on a break from studying, we picked through this care package and couldn't help but notice the large bunch of pills packed in aluminum foil and Bubble Wrap, held together by a rubber band and marked VICODIN. That evening, after reading in our pharmacology book how it caused extreme "euphoria and a false sense of well-being," we were destined to try it.

It was surprisingly difficult to pry the pills free from their casing, as if the physical barrier could protect against the incomparably seductive and alluring qualities of these pills. I started trying to gnaw one of the pills free, until Tami picked up scissors.

Thirty minutes after swallowing my first Vicodin, I felt a rapid rise of bliss in my heart, swelling to a state of happiness I had never known. It was better than Ecstasy. The word "euphoria" doesn't quite describe it. It is better described by William

Burroughs in *Junky* as "a way of life." A more accurate description would be: the beginning of the end.

Once the pills were gone, we settled back into the routine of medical school, with one change. As explained to me by Dr. Stern of SHP seventeen years later: "You've changed your brain forever." Far more than the Valium prescribed by Dr. Goldstein while I was at Greenpeace, trying Vicodin with Tami was a watershed event that had awakened the beast.

What this translated into was that some part of my brain, from that point on, was always on the lookout for pills, attempting to recreate my initial experience with Vicodin.

My next rotation was in the emergency department at Boston City Hospital, where we saw that the good citizens of Roxbury, and the rest of Boston, were busily shooting, clubbing, stabbing, maiming, strangulating, injecting, and poisoning one another, or themselves, or were driving under the influence or playing with explosives.

The medical complaint of most of the ER patients was usually in some way drug or alcohol related. Though I had started to form the habit of squirreling away whatever pills I happened across, to ingest them later, pills that, ironically, were chemically similar or identical to the drugs these people were abusing, I still dealt with these patients with condescending pity and sanctimony.

Their plight seemed entirely different from mine. I continued to view myself as part of the non-drug-taking medical establishment, successful, sober, responsible, while these patients were the diseased underbelly of our society. I had absolutely *nothing* in common with them.

One patient choreographed a complex imitation of a grand mal seizure in order to scam Valium, which was "the only thing that stops my seizures." She had done this before, and we all started clapping before she was finished, which surprised her enough to interrupt her "seizure" mid-thrash. Hallelujah! She's cured.

We laughed derisively about this "pseudoseizure" for weeks. If only I had known the lengths, later on, to which I would go for the same medication, or the misery I would experience when

I tested positive for it by Society to Help Physicians, then I might not have been so cocksure.

Another patient called me a "kike" and tried to kick me in the head when I told him we wouldn't be giving him any pain medications. Years later, I would understand what it was like to be dope sick, and why he was so violent.

A homeless woman, who had a severe pelvic infection from trading sexual favors for heroin, slurred out "I don't give a fuck" and then walked out when I told her it would be life threatening for her to leave without antibiotics. Years later, I would risk my health on drugs and ignore all but the most immediate consequences of my actions. But at the time, I had nothing in common with these losers.

Slowly, imperceptibly, as medical school went by, my seeking out, obtaining, and use of these medications escalated. As medical school was nearing a close, and we were busy applying to residency programs, I was in the habit of stealing meds from the nurses' stations, the supply closets of the different practices I rotated through, especially Orthopedics, which was always well-stocked, and from patients' rooms, if I saw them lying around unguarded.

I was losing control over the pills. I found some hydrocodone syrup in a supply closet at the community health center where I worked as a medical student. I swigged while still in clinic, and found my eyes drooping toward the end of our day's session. My preceptor was too distracted by her primary care patients to notice how out of it I was. This was such a close call, but I was still unable to stop myself.

The best part, from the viewpoint of a selfish addiction wishing to flourish, was that I was trusted and no one suspected me. I was under the radar.

As part of our Geriatrics rotation, we went on home visits to attend to patients who were homebound. Many of the apartments we visited were shabby, noisy, unsafe, and smelled terribly, like mold, urine, rotten garbage, and spoiled food. These apartments made the hellhole where I lived during medical school seem like the Ritz in comparison.

Part of our assignment during these home visits was to go through, sort, and organize the medications the patients were taking at home, to help them avoid confusion and duplication. I was now the wolf guarding the henhouse.

I would return from visits with my pockets full of pills. I started bringing empty, innocuously labeled bottles with me, which I could fill up, putting a piece of tissue paper in the bottle to muffle the sound of the pills bouncing around.

At the time, I didn't feel guilty, because I was helping people. Who cared if I skimmed a little off the top? I rationalized that my actions provided a net benefit. I was ever more desperate, because pills were rapidly becoming the only way to meet my increasingly neglected emotional needs. I was starting to suffer from withdrawal when the pills wore off. Necessity is the mother of invention, and I was taking greater risks.

Still, there was an upper limit, during my medical school years, to my access to prescription narcotics, which served as a rate-limiting step in the development of my addiction. There were only so many pills to encounter in a hospital setting. I was essentially a hunter-gatherer, relying on what I came across in my day-to-day clinical work, and occasionally supplementing this by searching the medicine cabinets of friends, colleagues, and relatives. My modus operandi was about to change, as I entered my residency and obtained prescription-writing privileges.

Due to some combination of idealism and masochism, I decided to pursue a residency in primary care. In spite of the drugs, my board scores were in the ninety-sixth percentile, and my dean's summary read as follows:

On behalf of Boston University School of Medicine, I am pleased to enthusiastically recommend Peter Grinspoon to you. Put simply and plainly, Peter is a star. He is keenly intelligent, mature, enthusiastic, highly motivated, and well-rounded. He has an outstanding fund of medical knowledge and has performed at the highest academic level throughout his entire four years. Hardworking and extremely conscientious, Peter functions exceptionally well as a member of the health care team. Compassionate and caring, Peter develops excellent rapport with his patients, far beyond that of his peers. His strong social conscience has kept him active in community and extracurricular activities throughout his medical education. I am pleased to recommend Peter Grinspoon as an outstanding candidate.

I was a "star" in med school because of the breadth of my experiences at Swarthmore and Greenpeace, and it's ironic that, partially because of Swarthmore and Greenpeace, I was now on drugs. I "matched" at the Brigham and Women's Hospital, one of Harvard's most prestigious, in their primary care program. At this point, I would have my own prescription pad.

Nate said, "Thanks for that thoughtful and honest overview, Charlie Brown...I mean Grinspoon. Really good work. I could even follow some of it, despite the big words. Do you ever confuse yourself?"

Three weeks into this introductory routine at Tannenberg, I graduated from living in Tannenberg Rehab itself to off-campus apartments in Wilson Village, which was nestled in a nearby, nondescript suburb, about a ten-minute drive away.

Wilson Village is made up of identical freestanding clusters of low-income apartments, decorated with sparse landscaping that was littered with trash, an artificial lake with a central fountain that spouted muddy water, and a run-down common area with some broken exercise machines and a nonfunctioning soda machine.

Our apartment had two bedrooms off the main room, which, economically, included both the living room and the kitchen. The rug was burnt orange, with tracks worn in it from the sofa to the bathroom. All of the furniture in the sitting room was oriented toward the central shrine of the television, which was always blaring and flickering. There was a small, cement porch sticking off the living room, littered with ash, with two plastic chairs and a tiny barbecue grill, and a low iron fence for decoration, or perhaps to keep you from crawling off the side if you were inebriated.

From the vantage point of this porch, I spent hours observing families go about their humdrum lives, with voyeuristic fascination. I felt guilty about the fact that, when my sentence of ninety days was up, I'd (hopefully) return to a life of material excess and intellectual privilege. My punishment for being addicted to drugs and for writing phony prescriptions was to reside temporarily in their permanent reality. It didn't seem fair. Their punishment for the same type of crime I committed, as poor members of a minority class, would be a long jail term.

Soon after my arrival at Wilson Village, there was a commotion outside. A semi, painted with the bright colors of Bud Light, had taken the off-ramp curve too quickly and had overturned across the way from us, disgorging hundreds of cases of beer onto a large triangular patch of grass. All of the alcoholics among us flocked to the window, like vampires watching a large spill of human blood just outside.

One of the vampires was my roommate James, an alcoholic, who spent whatever free time he had over the next few days longingly watching them clean up all the spilled beer. Just as the prisoners at Alcatraz were able to see the festive lights of San Francisco, but not participate in the festivity, James could watch this beer but not drink it, multiplying his misery.

James was in his midsixties, paunchy, graying, with a patronizing, professorial demeanor, which stemmed from the fact that he was certified in addiction medicine as well as internal medicine. All that knowledge about how to treat addiction in others didn't stop him from showing up at his addiction prevention clinic falling-down drunk.

James condescended to me, because he thought that being an alcoholic was less morally debased than being a drug addict. I had never met an elitist alcoholic before. His most painful habit was the white-noise machine, which he insisted on using at night to sleep. It created repetitive sounds of waves crashing into a beach, which, after several nights, started to influence my dreams. They began to take place in a beach or ocean setting.

My other roommate was Rudy, who remains to this day one of the most sociopathic people I have ever met. Short and wiry, with hair and teeth the color of the prison jumpsuit he was wearing just a few months earlier, he continually expelled cigarette smoke and misanthropy. The first thing he said to me, his idea of a joke: "How do you reason with a girl who has two black eyes? You can't, you've already tried twice." What could I say to this? I couldn't laugh at this disgusting joke, but I didn't feel like alienating my new roommate, or getting beaten.

Rudy instantly reminded me of prisoners I had helped take care of during medical school at Boston City Hospital. They got right into your face and had no respect for personal boundaries. Every interaction was a probing of your weaknesses, for any available way for them to take advantage of you. But at Boston City they usually had ankle chains, handcuffs, and at least two guards to control their behavior. They weren't free-range, cageless sociopaths like Rudy, free to act on the threat of physical violence they constantly communicated.

Rudy often boasted of having spent several years behind bars for felony assault convictions. I ignored most of his other nonsense as idle bragging, but this I believed. He had an explosive temper, and I shudder to imagine what he was like when drunk. I'd hate to be at the receiving end. He told me that in prison, he "fought dirty" by picking up the nearest chair and clubbing his opponent during fistfights.

Rudy was always asking me if he could borrow money, which he had no intention of repaying. For the first time, I started hiding my possessions in my car, so he couldn't steal them. Whenever anyone female said anything at all, he'd respond (if no supervisors were around), "If I want your opinion, I'll take my dick out of your mouth." Did he drive his cellmates nuts in prison, or were they all like this? Or did prison make him this way?

Rudy was responsible for most of the petty theft that occurred at the Tannenberg Rehab. He was usually broke in the morning and flush with cash by the afternoon. I knew this because, as roommates, we shopped together. Due to the no-solitude rule, we were together for the duration, and I spent half of my time waiting for a knife in my back, though he seemed to have identified me as harmless and vaguely entertaining.

Strange as my roommates were, Lyle's seemed even stranger. John, a farm boy from rural Tennessee, kidnapped a goat to raise drug money. I guess human beings have always used the tools available to them. "Have the goat bleat once into the phone if he is unharmed..."

Another patient was Butch, a surgeon from Massachusetts, who was well dressed and comported himself with the look of a busy and successful physician. This was a look that would prove to be no longer necessary. Butch had sold a scrip for Oxycontin to an undercover policeman. He was selling Oxycontin prescriptions to support his crack cocaine habit. He went straight from Tannenberg to jail, which he later described as "unbelievably anxiety provoking" and "not at all helpful to my recovery." He was a gentle soul, cut from a different cloth than Rudy, and wouldn't have survived much longer in prison.

At Wilson Village, our daily lives were similar to our days at Tannenberg, with the exception that, with longer leashes, we were able to go farther astray during the nighttime. It was impossible for the counselors to keep tabs on us. They were forced to rely on the "rat out your friends if they break the rules" rule, which didn't always work. If a group of people trusted one another, and had a common interest in not getting caught, no one would snitch.

One of our frequent destinations was mini golf, approved by the authorities as wholesome entertainment. We played marathon tournaments, alcoholics versus drug addicts. The addicts usually won because their hands were less shaky, though they didn't always hit the ball in the right direction. We didn't allow redos for hallucinations or double vision.

At that stage in my withdrawal, I had a difficult enough time keeping the ball on the green putting surface. I hadn't laughed this much since college, mostly at myself for putting the little yellow golf ball into low Earth orbit. It reminded me of playing mini golf with my twin brother as kids, when we would deliberately whack each other's ball over the highway, and end the game thirty seconds after we started.

The other common destination, which we were specifically instructed to avoid, was Hooters, a bar that features buxom young waitresses in tight white shirts and skintight neon-orange shorts.

The food at Hooters genuinely is good, especially the wings, and that was our pretext for going there. With pitchers of draft beer at every other table, and a full-length bar overflowing with any type of alcohol you could ask for, Hooters was the last place we should have been. I imagine that for an alcoholic, which accounted for about half of our group, eating dinner in a bar would be equivalent to my being in a pharmacy after-hours, with no supervision, or at a party with bowls of Percocets instead of hors d'oeuvres. Why tempt yourself?

The decor of the Hooters was largely dependent on pinups of bikini-clad models, and on the waitresses, who instantly greet you as if each of you is the guy they have always been waiting for and would love to hook up with. Like any bar, rock and roll was blasting in the background, and there were men and women in different stages of inebriation.

Our waitress, Candy, or Barbi, sported an improbably tight shirt imprisoning surgically augmented boobs, bleach-blonde hair, tight orange shorts that were the color of Rudy's teeth, or his prison jumpsuit, and what seemed to be several millimeters of makeup caked onto her face. I would have pegged her at sixteen years old.

In between her smiling, upbeat appearances at our table, she looked mostly sad and beaten down. My only contribution to the general testosterone- and bravado-filled conversation with her was when I asked her what she did when not working as a waitress, and she said, "Saving up so I can apply to college."

Lyle and I had different takes on Hooters. Because he had met his wife, Sandra, during a Hooters golf tournament, he argued in favor of Hooters: "It's harmless fun. It's a good way for a girl to make a living, and she don't even have to take off her clothes. The girls that work here are 'specially nice to the other girls that come in, so they feel comfortable. It's win-win for everybody."

That was a good argument, but personally, I thought Hooters was far more depressing than arousing. It seemed a watered-down version of the oldest profession, where men only got glimpses and women only got small change, like a melding of pornography and Muzak. It seemed degrading to all parties involved.

I'm sure it was worse for groupmate Adam in his gayness, having the entire evening oriented around having all his companions drool over a gender he wasn't interested in. When we returned from Hooters, Rudy would lock himself into the bathroom for hours. The rest of us were too afraid and disgusted to knock on the door and tell him to stop hogging the bathroom.

After about a month in rehab, when I started slowing down to a normal speed, and the medical staff were able to peel off some of my sedatives, I was told it was time for my psychological and cognitive testing. The psychologist reminded me of Mr. Spock, without the pointy ears, as he coldly and logically prodded me with questions.

His first question was, "Who painted the Sistine Chapel?" What's his name? Crap. I know this. It begins with an *M*. Italian. Renaissance. I should know this. I'm a doctor, dammit, not an encyclopedia. Maybe the drugs did hurt my memory.

"Time is up."
"Umm...Leonardo da Vinci?"

Wrong.

For several hours, he tested me on such things as how many numbers I could remember and repeat, forward and backward. He blindfolded me and had me try to fit shapes back into a vertical board that had holes cut out corresponding to these shapes. This was frustrating; I felt like I was flunking out of kindergarten.

He asked how many words I could come up with starting with an *F* in sixty seconds. Fake. Fickle. Feckless. Fantastic farting ferret food. Fenestrated fanlike featured failure. Frustrated. Farmaceuticals. And, of course, the F-word. I could have happily gone on all day. He had to stop me. On this particular subtest, Spock said that I produced 50 percent more words than the score that coincided with the ninety-ninth percentile.

He concluded that everything was basically functioning properly, though he wondered if I had manic tendencies, especially with all the *F* words. Brilliant deduction, Sherlock...I mean Spock. Anyone who has met me knows I have manic tendencies.

In group the next day: "Nate, did you know that I have manic tendencies? That's what the shrink says." Nate, who had by now suffered a whole month of my nervous energy, grandiosity, megalomania, and flights of ideas, rolled his eyes. "Grinspoon, you make Charlie Brown look like an intellectual. Sit still. You make me nervous. I liked you better on the sedatives. We know you hate to talk. Tell us about becoming a doctor, during your residency, and what it had to do with your addiction. We can't wait for the next episode. And, for God's sake, *speak slowly*, so the rest of us can follow."

I finished off my seventh cup of coffee that morning, took a few deep breaths, and launched in.

The first morning of medical residency at the Brigham did not go well. I couldn't wait to get the first day's jitters over with, and I was deeply focused on the tasks at hand: memorizing the charts of my new patients, introducing myself to them, writing my first orders for the nurses, and organizing my index cards so I could coherently present these patients to the team.

Around this time, I had heard from my parents that our close family friend Joel, a fixture of my childhood, was in the Brigham, dying of lung cancer. I made a mental note to visit him, but was preoccupied with this major transition, and it slipped my mind.

My first rotation was Oncology. The residents were assigned the Sisyphean task of trying to keep these patients comfortable and optimistic in the face of their chemotherapy-induced nausea, nerve pain, bleeding, sterility, and uncertain prognosis. We often had to wear masks and gloves to interact with them, because they had compromised immune systems, which diminished any human warmth or connection.

This whole routine forced me to imagine what Danny must

have gone through in the final weeks of his life, the doctors being nice to him, through masks and gloves, but also pulling back a little, knowing he was going to die.

On this first morning, during rounds, just as I started presenting my cases to our attending physician, a kind and avuncular if slightly intimidating prostate cancer specialist, I noticed several familiar faces congregated around the door of one of the patient rooms, just down the hall from where we were clustered. They looked stricken, and were hugging, crying, and clinging to one another. Putting this together, I surmised that our friend Joel had just passed away.

Witnessing this scene unfolding paralyzed me with confusion and indecision. At that moment, there were two competing frames of reference, each demanding my undivided attention. I couldn't "break rounds," having just started, being overawed by the immediate expectations of the team, and not wanting to miss any practical instruction on my first day in a new hospital. We were supposed to display a military level of discipline.

Equally, I couldn't ignore the heart-wrenching drama that was tugging at me from just down the hall, involving people I had known for decades.

With the expectant eyes of the team on me, I froze, midsentence, for a long, awkward minute, performed some quick mental calculations, and said, "I'm really sorry, a friend of my family just died, and I have to go deal with this." The attending was gracious and understanding when I returned twenty minutes later, shaken and distracted, after dealing with the grief-filled chaos of a deathbed situation.

This encounter, in the opening moments of my becoming a doctor, transformed my experience of patient care into something more real and human. After witnessing this death, not of a stranger but of a friend, as I was forming my first impressions, it was harder for me to retreat into the standard academic defenses that many doctors adopt to shield themselves. Instead of mere charts, names, and numbers, there were now real people, with families, attached to the patients I was caring for, who would hug one another and suffer if their loved one passed.

*   *   *

The bleakest rotation I went through during my residency was the Bone Marrow Transplant Unit, where entire immune systems would be wiped out with chemotherapy, and then replaced or regrown, on the slim chance that the patients, and not their cancer cells, would survive this profoundly toxic treatment.

As I was making rounds early one morning, I was dressed, as always when in the land of transplant, in gown, mask, and gloves, like some low-level worker from my visit to Chernobyl. I happened into the room of a patient I had met several times before, a very friendly and engaging eighteen-year-old who spent her time animatedly discussing what she was going to do when she had completed her bone marrow transplant, plans for hiking, travel, camping, dating, and college. She even had a pink package of birth control pills on the counter, anticipating a happier life.

On this particular morning, she had just been notified by our attending that her transplant was a failure, her cancer had survived, and there was nothing left to offer her. No one managed to communicate this to me before I blithely walked into her hospital room to wish her a hearty good morning.

What I walked into was a hurricane of fury, hopelessness, and destruction, a private moment of despair. Her face was distorted with pain and she was smashing everything in her room. She screamed, to no one in particular, "Fuck you, fuck you!" She looked at me but didn't recognize me. I beat a hasty, cowardly retreat and was shaking from more than just the caffeine when I left her room.

I didn't know how to process this, and I didn't have time to discuss it with anyone, because I had a whole sequence of patients to round on, and I couldn't keep the team waiting. That night, walking home, I was determined to get as high as possible to blot out the memory of this awful tragedy, which reminded me so much of Danny. I was aiming for pure obliteration.

After thirty-six-hour shifts, I would try to clear my mind by walking home, which took forty-five minutes, to the second-story apartment I shared with my betrothed, H. Ignoring the smog from the car-infested Jamaicaway, I settled into the rhythm of my footsteps and allowed the stress of the previous night to dissipate. I replayed the scenes and struggles in my mind, wondering what I could have done differently and second-guessing many of my treatment decisions. I would also plot my drug use for the next several hours.

Not having seen me for two days, H. would naturally be bored and lonely, craving conversation and affection or, depending on her mood, conflict and drama. After these long shifts, I didn't have anything left. Even if our relationship hadn't been showing early signs of strain, I was empty: physically, mentally, emotionally, and spiritually. It was useless trying to get anything out of me. I often had blistering headaches.

The last thing I was equipped to deal with at this point was H.'s mood swings, and I absolutely, positively didn't want to deal with the long list of chores that she would compile for me in my absence. If I wasn't a passive doormat by nature, and too tired to fight, I would have said, "I've been working for thirty-six hours. You do your own dishes."

Instead, as soon as possible, I would crash hard, falling into a deep, dreamless, drugged sleep. I wouldn't even pause to brush my teeth before falling asleep.

I facilitated my fall into unconsciousness with pills and with pot, sneaking onto our back porch to smoke; anything to become blissfully unconscious, free of worries, tuned out from life, with its stress, guilt, and conflict, its responsibilities and disappointments. I would seek obliteration, nothingness. No dreams, just darkness.

Twelve hours later, seemingly in the blink of an eye, it was time to head back to the hospital. Sorry, H., time to go. I'll get to those dishes next time. Duty calls.

The time I spent out of the hospital started to take on a surreal, dreamlike quality of its own. My outside life was completely separate from the alternate reality I lived in the hospital, and I felt that I was getting it from both ends; work was stressful and exhausting, and my home life was conflictual and equally exhausting.

The only untainted time I had to myself was my forty-five-minute walk home from the hospital, where, as if in a magical buffer zone, I was unclaimed by the demands of either world. Some days I wished I could keep walking but never arrive.

Against this background of long shifts, sleep deprivation, emotionally challenging clinical scenarios, depressing rotations, and the loneliness of a disillusioning relationship at home, it was increasingly difficult to resist the draw of the pills I encountered in the hospital, in patients' rooms, in clinics, and in supply closets. These were a quick fix for my increasingly neglected emotional needs.

I didn't have any extra time or energy to worry about the fact that I was taking pills almost every day. I always filed away this problem for later consideration, and promised myself that, once life slowed down a little, I'd get a handle on it. It was on my to-do list, next to making an appointment with the dentist. It was the same thing with the warning signs in my relationship with H.: When I have some time and some rest, I'll deal with this, but definitely not right now, when I'm feeling so overwhelmed.

Taking pills was a way of saying "fuck you" to the unreasonable demand that I stay up all night in the hospital, to H. for being so controlling, to the eighteen-year-old for dying of cancer, not to mention an extra fuck you for Danny, for the trees that are being cut down, and for my weird upbringing, which didn't include Little League or any normal activities. It was my Greenpeace-like protest against whatever there was in my life that I was unhappy about.

For all of us newly minted medical interns, it was a power trip to be able to prescribe medications on our own, without the cosignature of a supervisor. After years of medical school, countless exams and hours of study, endless drudgery and abuse on our clinical rotations, and hundreds of thousands down the drain in tuition, we had finally become little gods with the godlike ability to prescribe medications. This was our just reward, part of doctor eminent domain, something we felt fully entitled to.

With gusto, we prescribed each other penicillin for sore throats and steroid creams for rashes. It was only a matter of time until I crossed the next line in the sand, my personal Pandora's box, the line that, ultimately, would precipitate my spectacular downfall as a physician and land me in the deepest of shit. I started experimenting with the limits of my prescription pad.

At the time, nobody suspected that giving me a prescription pad was like giving a book of matches to a pyromaniac, or an atomic bomb to a terrorist. As I was to discover over the next several years, with just a pen and a small, square piece of paper, and the exertion of a few scribbles, I could transport my mood (Percocet, Vicodin), provide myself with inexhaustible energy (uppers), or hasten my disappearance into the land of oblivion (Valium and Klonapin), at will and with ease.

My prescription pad potentially offered a vastly higher yield than my hunter-gatherer method of pill collection. In theory, with this pad and the knowledge of how to make prescriptions happen, in my name or borrowing a colleague's name, or the name of a patient, a friend, or a relative, my access to pills was limited only by my need to remain undetected and to keep up appearances at work and in my home life.

The first time it occurred to me to write a spurious prescription was, symbolically enough, on my honeymoon with H. in Maine, which occurred at the end of my internship year. After our wedding, a beautiful outdoor affair at the rustic Paine Estate in Waltham, Massachusetts (also thought of by me now as the House of Pain), we drove up to Eastport, Maine, staying in various decorous bed-and-breakfasts, eating lobster in the rough on the rocky seashore, walking on the beach, and visiting bookstores and coffee shops.

On paper, it was bliss, except that, in reality, I was suffering from migraines, I had a skin infection on my leg, and I was feeling bored and restless. As our physical intimacy diminished, I was wondering if I had just made a fateful mistake. I was utterly fried both from residency and the wedding I had just weathered.

It didn't occur to me until years later that the reason I was feeling so antsy and uncomfortable was that I was withdrawing. This was the first time since residency began that I was away from the hospital for more than a few days, and it was the first time that I didn't have regular access to the pills I would obtain in the hospital. I didn't realize or notice that I had been taking pills most days. This level of use sort of snuck up on me.

I wouldn't have noticed it for a day or two, but now that I was off meds for more than a week, it was hitting me like a ton of bricks.

This feeling of escalating jitteriness was threatening to subsume the relaxing and romantic aspects of my honeymoon. I was shaky and sweaty, and this is hard to hide. I had not thought to bring any pills or pot with me, assuming that I would be relaxed away from the hospital on my honeymoon. H. repeatedly asked me what was wrong, but I couldn't very well say to her, "I need drugs, and I'm in withdrawal." That wouldn't have set the right tone for the rest of our marriage.

Several days into this, I was off for a solitary walk on the beach, hoping to work off some of my jitters, while H. was antique shopping. My mind wandered back to the subject of the pills I wasn't taking. As I turned back into town, I came across a pharmacy on one side of the street and a payphone on the other.

It suddenly occurred to me that I could phone the pharmacy up in the guise of another doctor calling in a prescription for Peter Grinspoon. I could feel better immediately, improve my honeymoon, and get my marriage started off on the right foot. Where was the harm in this? To my twisted thinking, it was a win-win situation.

Somewhat nervous with anticipation, just as I felt at age twelve, smoking marijuana for the first time on the beach on Cape Cod, I entered the phone booth and dialed the pharmacy across the street from me. They must not have had caller ID or they might have noticed I was calling from the same area code, from just across the street.

"Hello, this is Dr. Sadistky calling from Boston. I'm calling in a prescription for Soma (a loosely controlled muscle relaxant/ barbiturate) for patient Peter Grinspoon." Half an hour later, I casually walked in and retrieved this prescription, and proceeded to have a relaxing honeymoon, marveling at what a brilliant, Greenpeace-seasoned criminal mastermind I was. What a lethal precedent this set for my nascent medical career.

Did I mention that Pandora's box was open?

My summary recommendation from my residency program at the Brigham reads as follows:

> Peter is an outstanding clinician who has been extraordinarily effective in taking care of his clinic patients. He is highly intelligent and knowledgeable. He forms caring relationships with his patients and has made a significant difference in the lives of many of them. He is able to connect with hard-to-reach patients and is patient and persevering in getting his patients to make important lifestyle changes... The successful clinical outcomes in his patient panel are the result of his superb relationships with his patients and his dedication to their well-being...Peter is also a highly effective and caring teacher...Most important, Peter is a wonderful person and, consequently, a wonderful colleague. He is idealistic, kind, generous and has great integrity...He is an outstanding team player...In summary, Peter is a gem. His intelligence, kindness and communication skills make him highly effective as a clinician, teacher and colleague.

Reading that I had "great integrity" made me feel false and guilty. There must have been at least some integrity left, in the part that wasn't yet corroded by the drugs. My face burned in shame when I thought, "What if they knew what I'm really up to?"

Toward the end of residency, I was developing cracks in my facade, either from the drugs or from sheer burnout and exhaustion. I started to let my clinical work slide. I would freeze up in complex situations, such as during codes, when we had to resuscitate patients. I stopped participating in anything that wasn't absolutely required. I didn't even go to the resident dinner where they had a whole skit about how hyper and neurotic I was. I crawled over the finish line.

With glazed eyes, Nate said, "That was dizzying, Grinspoon. Truly dizzying. Not just because of the big words. Doctors have very unique risks and susceptibilities to addiction. They have the access and the stress. We'll continue to discuss these themes you brought up, once the headache you've given me goes away."

During our next didactic section, Nate moved on to the current topic, which was that "addiction is a brain disease." This way of thinking about addiction espouses the idea that much or most of a person's addiction is due to their intrinsic brain chemistry, certain neurotransmitters predominating over others, which is why we crave and seek out drugs.

Yay! It's not my fault. Blame it on my brain, all of it. My brain stole the drugs. My brain wrote those bad scrips. I'm just an innocent corpse, hostage to this evil, drug-seeking brain. My brain has a mind of its own. This is my brain on drugs. My *brain* is on drugs. Set me free from this rogue brain.

I was ready to start kneeling in celebration with Zeke the coal miner. I was ready to face the judge as well as the medical board. They would drop the criminal charges and restore my medical license promptly, once I sat them down and gave them an edifying lecture on addiction as a brain disease, and how none of this was remotely my fault. They might even apologize for the misunderstanding.

Nate rapidly burst my bubble. "Calm down, Grinspoon. They are still going to put your ass in a sling. And throw away the key. Though sometimes, if the judge is smart, he might consider other factors. Medical boards don't view it this way at all. As doctors, they should, but they will nail you."

One of Nate's main challenges was to keep us focused in the present, and to ensure that we were truly in rehab, being rehabilitated, so that we wouldn't repeat the same mistakes upon our return home. This wasn't (just) a prison sentence; it was supposed to fix me, which required, more than anything else, being in the here and now. I couldn't benefit from therapy if I spent the time worrying and daydreaming (or daynightmaring) about my return to Boston.

I was utterly panicked about the horrific thicket that was awaiting me in Boston, which loomed closer as each day passed. Daily, I received notification, sometimes by certified mail or FedEx, of some new sanction from the DEA, an HMO, one of the health insurance companies, my disability company, my hospital, the American Board of Internal Medicine, or my malpractice carrier. Not to mention H. and her threats and my uncertain status at home. Or the criminal charges.

Conferring with Solomon over the phone about my status with the medical board, I began to understand that any potential return to work was a shifting goal line, and that it wasn't absolutely guaranteed. First it had looked like three months, then six. "They want a certain amount of time with you clean and sober before they even consider a return to work. They likely will want to see twelve months of clean time. They don't like that you involved patients in your addiction."

What? A year? What will happen to my patients? How are we going to afford this? Had I known then that it was going to be almost four years before I returned to work, I would have simply given up.

Swamped with remorse, I also kept revisiting the past. How could I steal drugs? How could I lie to all those kind people who trusted me? Will my friends, colleagues, and family forgive me? Will they ever trust me again? Will anyone? Would any of the patients with whom I shared drugs try to sue me? I'd get slaughtered in a lawsuit. Would they try to blackmail me? (Blackmailing occurs more often than one would think. An addicted patient can say, "Continue to prescribe my drugs or I report you to the medical board." I've seen this happen on several occasions.)

In May 2002, when I started my new job at Boston's Faulkner Hospital, a well-respected community hospital in the Jamaica Plain neighborhood, adjacent to the Arnold Arboretum, I was desperately hoping to have a fresh start. But my addiction stowed away in the boxes I brought containing my stethoscope, diplomas, textbooks, and medication samples. It made itself at home in my new practice life.

Within a few weeks, my new desk became littered with charts, lab results, medication samples, coffee cups, papers to be filled out, phone messages, and medical magazines such as the *New England Journal of Medicine*. I couldn't quite keep up with this stuff, in addition to the steady stream of patients through my exam rooms and all the other demands on my time.

One feature of this practice was its deluxe medicine closet, which was stocked with pills for lower cholesterol and a smaller prostate, as well as antidepressants, migraine medications, and Viagra. This long, narrow room had a door that closed. No one could tell that I was inside.

Being inside this closet was a source of comfort for me, a secluded, peaceful cave, sort of like the black light room we had as kids with Danny. I spent quite a bit of time in there browsing or, rather, communing with the medications, feeling their energy, embracing their essence. I was slipping deeper into my addiction. I wasn't yet using every day, but I was feeling more and more of an irresistible allure from these drugs.

At work, I was starting to fray around the edges. Several times a day, I would go for walks in between patients and smoke cigarettes, wearing latex gloves and chewing gum so I wouldn't reek when I got back. Patients still smelled it and complained.

I started seeing a psychiatrist. During one session with her, I was uncharacteristically honest. "I'm completely miserable, at home and at work. Percocet is the only thing that makes me happy. Can you write me a prescription for sixty pills?"

She passed on pursuing this further, ignoring a red flag that could be seen from space—a doctor admitting absolute dependence on an opiate to improve his mood. She said, "That is out of the bounds of conventional treatment," and let it go at that. I wonder what my life might have been like had she chosen to intervene at that point.

One of the first patients I met at this new job was Cindy, a twenty-five-year-old graduate student in sociology, very tall, with red hair, a warm smile, but cold, calculating eyes. Her frail body was wasted from the cystic fibrosis she had struggled with since early childhood.

Cindy's major symptoms were a cough, shortness of breath, and rib pain from constantly hacking, for which she was on a huge dose of methadone, a powerful narcotic, which is used to get people off heroin, but which is also used for pain control. She was changing doctors because her previous PCP was in trouble with the medical board for a narcotics violation.

Cindy had a seductiveness about her that was not physical. Somehow she drew me into her confidence. We seemed to recognize each other on some direct, subconscious level, druggie manipulator to druggie opportunist. She made veiled references to her dad and his role in organized crime, and to her mom sometimes taking her pills, both of which would have been warning signals if I had been functioning properly.

On the surface, she seemed sincere and innocent, and came across as the vulnerable underdog. During her inpatient hospitalizations, she wore pajamas and cuddled with a teddy bear. This was hardly my image of a sophisticated narcotics sociopath.

Soon after I assumed her care, she and I came to an arrangement where I would prescribe her two hundred fifteen pills of methadone instead of the two hundred she had been taking, and she would give me fifteen of them every month. We pretended she was an innocent friend/patient, helping out with my "migraines."

I can't remember the details of how this came about, it's blurry, but we were in conspiracy from the start, and I remember her laying her pills of methadone on my desk, essentially, nonverbally, offering them to me. We'd count out my fifteen pills together. It can't possibly be a coincidence that her previous doc, too, was in trouble for the same type of narcotics violation.

None of this is to say that this disgusting boundary violation wasn't entirely, absolutely my fault and my responsibility. She was the patient, and I had power over her. She needed the pills, though I'm still not certain for what legitimate use, and I used this to my advantage.

In making this Faustian bargain with Cindy, and about four

other patients, over the next two years, I crossed the third and final line in my descent. First, hunting and gathering (aka stealing). Next, fraudulently prescribing medication, which would lead, as I was to learn the hard way, to felony-level criminal violations. Now, worse, I was colluding with my most scheming, addicted, and criminal patients, to supply both their habits and mine.

There were some lines I didn't cross. I never robbed a pharmacy at knifepoint, wearing a balaclava. I never mugged little old ladies or stole their purses. I never kidnapped a goat and held it for ransom. I never shared needles or injected drugs. I never pimped, like some of my patients do, or hustled, like Robert Mapplethorpe in Patti Smith's *Just Kids*. I never dealt in street drugs like William Burroughs in *Junky*. I never became an unrecognizable animal, like David in Abraham Verghese's *The Tennis Partner*. I didn't live on the streets like Nic in *Beautiful Boy*. I didn't become paranoid and psychotic like Bill Clegg in *Portrait of an Addict as a Young Man*.

But seriously, how low can one go? With sick alchemy, I had transformed the dignity of being a doctor into the role of a highly educated pusher, exploiting my power, violating boundaries, and making a mockery of the "do no harm" clause of the Hippocratic oath. I was exploiting the very patients I was charged with healing.

Being in rehab while your life is melting down is like trying to focus on practicing the piano when the house around you is engulfed in flames. Every atom wants to call the fire department, spray the fire extinguisher, put a wet cloth over your mouth, and run outside with your favorite possessions, or at least your diary. All the while, your piano instructor is telling you to ignore the fire and play the song through to the end. Nate yanked me back to the present: "I'll advocate for you professionally, later, if (and only if) you stay in the here and now and do the work you need to do."

"Fine, Nate, but how am I going to pay for Tannenberg?" H.

had frozen all of our joint accounts. I saw at least one patient who couldn't pay her bill ruthlessly kicked to the curb by the for-profit bottom line at rehab. H. had decided it was my parents' fault that I was an addict, and insisted that they should have to pay any associated costs. I couldn't ask my parents to pay when H. and I had tons of money in the bank, accumulated from my workaholism.

It was difficult to know where I stood with H., because she seemed to be of two minds. My phone conversations with her were utterly unpredictable, sometimes civil, even affectionate. She started to discuss my coming home for a visit and her coming down for the family weekend. Words like "healing" and "together" would sneak into the conversation.

These conversations took place while, secretly, she was freezing the bank accounts.

Other conversations were less encouraging. "If you come back, you won't come back here, you won't see the kids until you are three months sober. Your exposure to the kids will be once a week. I'm taking the children to a therapist that specializes in custody and addiction issues."

We could have both types of conversations within the course of a few hours.

This ambivalence, or, more accurately, the split personality of this phase of our relationship, mirrors a fiercely contested ideological battle, which H. and I had been locked in for years, over who and what was to blame for the deterioration of our marriage.

To any and all, even to people who hardly knew us and didn't care, H. claimed that we would be a paradigm of nuptial harmony and bliss if it weren't for my drug use. She preached this with a religious fervor, analogous to that of the early Christians who risked dismemberment by hordes of barbarians but who zealously carried the faith nonetheless. Conveniently, this interpretation absolved her of any responsibility and put her in the role of the victim.

I'm not discounting the effects of my addiction or trying to wiggle out of my contributions to our marital meltdown, especially as time goes on and I'm able to look back on my foolish behavior.

But I thought our problems ran much deeper than the addiction. Too often, H. was all about spousal control and punishment, and about impressing the neighbors at the expense of her loved ones. She could be verbally abusive. To me, the addiction was in part a symptom of a deeper disharmony in our marriage.

During our marriage, my main refuge from our troubles, and from my work, was my diary, where I could explain, vent, record, and process. After I wrote my troubles down, they weighed less. This diary was like the fifth lobe of my brain. It was the one area of space in our home, in our lives, that I had carved out and defended for myself. I didn't hide it that well, because I naively thought that privacy would be universally respected.

My references to H. weren't always complimentary, because I was furious at her. She punished me, and withheld affection if I didn't do what she wanted. From where I stood, her view of marriage was that she was a feudal lord. She screamed so loudly, it's a wonder that our entire neighborhood doesn't have permanent hearing loss. She tried to control every aspect of my life.

For her part, she was furious about the pills, and to be honest, I can't imagine anything worse than an addicted spouse, slowly failing before your eyes, your dreams shattered, the person you loved not there anymore, disappearing piece by piece. It's impossible to bring up kids with someone who's not entirely present or reliable, though it's a good question which one of us was more reliable at that point. I was addicted, and she was crazed with anger.

One day, a few weeks before my departure for rehab, during a particularly savage fight, H. walked right over to the bottom drawer of my clothes closet, grabbed my diary without bothering to pretend to look for it, and locked herself in the bathroom. For me, this was the Apocalypse.

Secrets of my drug use were in there; I'd be caught red-handed. The jig would be up. My references to her were vicious; I referred to her as an "idiot bitch" and described elaborate escape fantasies that included divorce. She was trampling the last shred of my privacy, and putting a match to gunpowder at the same time.

I had to recover my diary before irreversible damage had been done. I have never been so single-minded. Through the door: "H., you have to give this back right away. This is unacceptable." "I'm busy." Her voice was calm, almost taunting. A bad sign. I could hear her scribbling away. She was annotating my diary with responses to my statements, like "that's nice" and "if you really don't want to be with me you don't have to."

Without thinking, I kicked in the bathroom door, splintering the wood where the lock had been attached, and ripped my diary out of her hands. From that point on, our marriage was utterly devoid of trust. Symbolically enough, I hid my diary in my car, where it could easily be evacuated from the marriage.

I brought my dilemma about whether my marriage was going to survive to Nate, who said, "Stop torturing yourself trying to intellect'lyze this out. The only way to tell what is her stuff and what is yours is to go back sober and healthy, set good limits, and see what happens. If it's better, blame the addiction. If it's worse, it's her stuff, you can't fix it, and it's time to move on." More prophetic words were never uttered.

But what about my Annie and Milo, whom I missed more than I'd ever missed anything? I wasn't free to just walk out on them. I know this isn't a great reason to stay with someone, but I didn't want to lose daily access to them. I've always been skeptical of the argument "Stay together for the kids." Who needs to grow up with parents who are constantly at each other's throats? They were all I had left.

I was desperate to avoid being one of those divorced dads you often see having awkward conversations with their small children, across the table from them in restaurants, the kids forced to act like little adults, sit still in a chair, and think of things to talk about. My working assumption was that it was worth putting up with an almost infinite amount of abuse from H. in order to retain the privilege of seeing them every day.

As it stood, in rehab, I wasn't entirely sure when I would see

Annie and Milo again, or even if they would remember me in more than just a superficial sense, as more than a friendly, sad shadow that they scribble notes to and occasionally speak with on the phone.

Ninety days is usually the recommended duration for doctors at rehab. That is a lifetime for a five-year-old and a four-year-old. Sometimes several more months of aftercare are encouraged by the counselors. I didn't have any choice but to abide by their recs. (It seemed to me that coal miners miraculously get cured in two or four weeks, because they can't pay as much. At for-profit rehab centers, the "clinical assessment" of how long a patient needed to remain in rehab often coincided uncannily with the patient's socioeconomic status and ability to pay. It feels like a racket.)

Even if I finished up in ninety days and returned right to Boston, it wasn't clear what access I would have to the kids, or where I would be living.

While I was away, my contact with the kids was completely dependent on H. It was intermittent at best, and tended to mirror her mood and disposition toward me. On good days, she would encourage them to talk on the phone with their cherished father, who would soon be healthy and join them again in a happy home. On bad days, I would hear nothing. This must have been as confusing to the kids as it was to me.

Annie and Milo frequently sent me cards decorated with crayon, scribbled with the words "get well soon." But, at ages five and four, they weren't proficient phone talkers. A typical phone conversation:

"Hi, Annie. Hi, Milo. How are you?"
"Good, Daddy."
"What have you been doing?"
"Talking to you on the phone."
"I miss you and I can't wait to see you."
"We miss you too, Daddy."
"I love you."
"We love you too, Daddy."

"Good-bye, Annie. Good-bye, Milo."

"Good-bye, Daddy. Daddy, we are going to hug and kiss the phone now."

Then I'd hear kisskisskisskiss, followed by H.'s grating, bitter voice in the background and a final click. I'd hold the receiver for a few minutes, still warm to my ear, while the echoes of their voices, and whatever temporary connection I had with them, died away.

These conversations left me feeling more alone and farther away. At one point, Annie said, "If you don't come home right now, I'll start to cry. I'm going to cry if you don't come home sooner." You and me both. When I called Milo to wish him a happy birthday, he said, "My birthday isn't really until you come home." Having had my birthday just a month earlier, I knew what he meant.

The worst part is that I felt I had brought all of this down upon them. Nate said my only recourse was to "focus on getting your own house in order so you can help them."

After ten weeks at rehab, the time came for my weekend-long home visit, a recovery "stress test" before permanent reentry. I was desperate to see my kids but nervous about dealing with H., not knowing what our status was and how she would react to my presence. The last few times we had been together didn't go so well.

The Tannenberg staff encouraged me to confront the chaos, triggers, shame, and judgment that awaited me back home, as well as any drugs I still had stashed around the house, with the opportunity to then return to the Tannenberg womb to process these experiences and to prove I could stay sober.

According to Nate, "You flunk [a drug test] when you get back here, you start over. If you find anything at home, flush it quick, and think about dealing with me after a positive test." I'd rather deal with an attack helicopter than with Nate after a positive test.

Going home seemed to bring all of my guilt and embarrassment to the forefront.

I was planning to stay with my parents, but H. invited me

back home for the weekend. She was lonely, and had a backlog of chores that needed to get done. I was desperate to reconnect with the kids, and affection-starved, so I swallowed my doubts, and my pride, and decided to chance it at the marital home. On some level, I knew that H. was Lucy, the kids were the football, and I was, once again, to play the part of Charlie Brown.

Nate encouraged me by pointing out that this was an ideal opportunity to go home, with all I was learning about myself, with the scales of oxycodone removed from my eyes, and to get a glimpse at whether my marriage could stay afloat. Nate's parting words of advice: "Grinspoon, don't ferget, you've changed a lot recently; they haven't."

Picking me up at Logan Airport, H. was civil, though we were tentative and awkward, like eighth-graders on our first date. Were we friends? Reconciled? Lovers? Soon to be divorced? Was I a little bit forgiven? I wondered if I was going through the motions of an attempted reconciliation with her because I wanted to be with her, or if it was just a Trojan horse to let me remain in close proximity to my kids. Nate's voice in my head told me to stop thinking so much. (Actually, it told the thinking part of my mind to "shut the fuck up.")

From the airport, we drove through the labyrinthine streets of Boston to retrieve Annie and Milo from the Allandale Farm camp, near to where we originally had met for our first date, in Jamaica Plain, seven years earlier, over coffee.

Allandale Farm, "Boston's last working farm," is an oasis in a suburban area between Brookline and Jamaica Plain, adjacent to the Faulkner Hospital, where I first encountered Bruno and Rufus. I instinctively shrank in my seat as we drove past, as if all of my former colleagues were waiting by the window for me to drive by, in order to gawk, cluck, and criticize.

Allandale hosts a small farm stand, rudimentary, just one room attached to greenhouses, where you can buy fresh produce and assorted yuppie delicacies. Adjacent to the farm stand, from what looks like an underground nuclear bunker, the camp lets out for the day. Annie and Milo, caked in mud, knowing that I would be there, bolted out, looking all around for me.

I saw them first and was struck by how, after ten weeks, they looked different, older, and alien, yet still the same, exactly the same, small and vulnerable. Beneath the smiles, I could see sadness and stress etched on their faces. They deserved better than this.

They recognized me and sprinted over. Annie is not athletic, but this could have been an Olympic qualifying sprint. Skinny for her age, with brown hair and incandescent blue eyes, she was wearing her purple raincoat, and I remember her flying leap into my arms, latching on to me as hard as her small arms would allow. We were both crying. Then Milo, with his curly blond hair, took his own flying leap and joined the scrum.

Life at home approximated normalcy, as if we were transported to an earlier time when we were just a family, without all of these tragic undercurrents. H. was frisky and playful, on her best behavior, as though she were the one on trial, and Annie and Milo couldn't have been happier to have their dad back in the picture.

We picnicked at the Arnold Arboretum, that vast oasis of greenery in the center of working-class Boston. This is the same arboretum that my office looked out over, until they locked me out of it forever. Annie ate cheese sticks, Milo ate a bagel with peanut butter, which dripped down his Thomas the Tank Engine shirt, and H. and I feasted on sandwiches that we constructed from gourmet ingredients purchased at the nearby ethnic markets.

"H., it's nice to be back and to reconnect. I'm sorry for all the fighting and for all of my screwups. I'm really trying to get better, and to work through all of this stuff."

"I missed you too, but you better not start using again. This is your last chance."

At home, there were reminders of my drug use everywhere I looked. I still had marijuana and paraphernalia hidden away in our back porch. I knew I should follow Nate's advice and dispose of it, but a subconscious, invisible hand prevented this. I left it there undisturbed, after giving it a nostalgic sniff. I didn't encounter any stashes of pills.

During this visit, I was vividly reminded of the sequence of events that got me busted in the first place, which brought all of this mess raining down on me.

One morning, in September of 2003, I developed an increasingly intense headache. It started out like one of my "migraines"—a minor headache that I milked and exaggerated to justify painkillers. It actually became a migraine but, oddly, on both sides of my head. I was the boy who cried wolf, so no sympathy or pain medication was allowed by H. who, by that time, had become deeply skeptical of any of my requests for medicine. (This is another good reason not to become a drug addict: When you genuinely need painkillers, no one is going to give them to you.)

The pain became blinding, so I discreetly asked my neighbor Greg for some Vicodin, which he was happy to provide, because with a recent letter I had supported his disability claim. To my dismay, this didn't touch the pain. Something was wrong. When I started throwing up and becoming frantic and irrational, H. dropped me off at the ER of the closest hospital, where I work.

Just inside the door, I sank to my knees in the lobby, barfed all over the rug, and slumped down on the floor in the middle of my mess. This is an excellent way to get prompt care in an emergency room.

Within the first hours after my arrival, the medical staff threw all sorts of tests at me: blood tests, urine tests, X-rays, and a CT scan. When suffering from meningitis, the last thing you want is to be poked and prodded. Even the smallest sounds made my head explode. An injection of Demerol, a powerful opiate, mildly blunted the pain.

It is routine to check toxicology screens in patients who present with severe headaches, to make sure the problem isn't coke or meth. Had they checked, my urine would have lit up like a Christmas tree. Pot, check. Vicodin, check. Oxycodone, check. Valium, check. Klonapin, check. They would have been forced to report me to the medical board, which would have forced me to get help. This might have stopped my life from imploding more than a year before it imploded.

They suggested doing a spinal tap, where they stick a needle into your back, directly into your spinal canal, suck out spinal fluid, and determine if there is an infection. I know, from having performed these in residency, that the pain goes to eleven. I tried to pull rank. "You need to stop overtreating me because I am a doctor. Just make this pain go away, so I can go home." They were not cowed at all. The last thing these battle-ax nurses cared about was the censure of a physician.

I was transported to my room by gurney, which bumped on corrugated metal ridges by the patient elevator. This hurt so much my vision flickered. My skull felt as if someone were cutting through it with a buzz saw (as I had done to my cadaver in medical school). I told myself, "If my patients can survive this, I can survive this." I remained in the hospital for eight days.

For the first three days, I barfed all over my room. I felt guilty that the orderlies had to keep mopping it up. I apologized profusely. It was difficult, waiting passively for someone to bring food or medicine. I was tethered to an intravenous. I didn't know what day it was. The experience of being in the hospital was as if a sadistic group of psychologists had set up a study of learned helplessness. I could see why my elderly people get disoriented. I could barely remember my name.

Being at my hospital of employment was a two-edged sword. Now that I was out of the ER, the nurses gave me VIP treatment, and my colleagues, mostly Dr. Hutch, my medical director, checked in on me every day. I was so sick, I wanted to crawl under a rock, lick my wounds alone, and avoid the social niceties that go with having visitors. Easier to be anonymous, unknown, and unaccountable.

Straining my ears, I could hear the medical team, rounding in the hallway, discussing my case. The senior resident lectured, "In an opiate-naive patient, we use a low dose, and that's usually all that's necessary to curb their pain without side effects." I was screaming in my head, "I'm not opiate naive! I take opiates every day! I'll die if you give me a very low dose." I couldn't bring myself to admit this to them.

My pain was managed by a device next to my bed which provided PCA or "patient-controlled analgesia." When in pain, I was instructed to press a red button, and that would trigger a small dose of pain medication into my intravenous. If pressed too frequently, it beeped loudly and locked you out until a certain amount of time had passed. This beep was excruciating, and caused me to press the button even more frequently, which caused more beeping...

Unable to complain without incriminating myself, I had to suffer through meningitis with a beginner's dose of Dilaudid. I cursed myself for getting into this mess, and resolved, again, to break free.

In September of 2004, five months before my encounter with Bruno and Rufus, I walked into the living room of our home in Hyde Park, and immediately noticed that something wasn't right with our au pair. Ruth, a tall, comely, live-in nanny from New Zealand, ordinarily upbeat and energetic, was lying on the sofa, bent over, clutching her stomach. She looked flushed, feverish, and she winced in pain when I pressed on the right lower side of her abdomen. Appendix? We rushed her to the Faulkner Hospital.

After her appendectomy, Ruth was discharged without any pain medications, a common oversight in the hustle and bustle of hospital life, by oblivious and goal-directed surgeons. As a doctor, and as a concerned host parent, I felt obligated to prescribe something for her discomfort. Ruth didn't drive, so I drove her to the pharmacy. It pained her to walk, so I left her in the car while I picked up her prescription.

Performing these two activities together, prescribing and picking up, gave my addiction-addled brain a sudden inspiration: Why involve the patient at all? Oh joy! The perfect crime! Ruth would soon be back in New Zealand. How could it possibly hurt her if I prescribed in her name and picked it up for her? How could it hurt anyone, except for the evil insurance companies who should pay more anyway? (Answer: Several months later, Ruth would be questioned by the police in New Zealand, as part of the criminal investigation into my prescribing. This was terrifying to her.)

For the immediate future, this new idea solved my supply problems.

This scam would have succeeded once or twice, with several months in between. Prescription-wise, there was nothing ostensibly out of the ordinary about it. Thousands of prescriptions get written every day, hundreds by my office alone. How would the pharmacist know that Ruth wasn't taking these pills? Or that she was out of the country?

A desperate criminal is not a careful criminal. I was slipping deeper in, which limited my ability to critically evaluate terrible ideas. My various schemes were not meticulously planned and executed Greenpeace actions, but a series of impulsive, risky behaviors. "Ruth" went through several prescriptions for Vicodin in rapid succession. "Ruth" even had a prescription for Suboxone, the medication that Dr. T. prescribed for me to wean me off opiates. I didn't even have the special license that is needed to prescribe Suboxone.

It is no wonder that the pharmacist became suspicious. She phoned me on my cell, the number I left with the prescription the first time I dropped it off. "Hello, this is the pharmacist from CVS calling. Is Ruth there?" Panic. How was I supposed to answer this? Maybe in New Zealand, Ruth is a gender-neutral name like Pat or Jean.

"Ummmm...speaking."

"Ruth, we are trying to confirm some information. Can you please confirm your birthday?"

Checkmate. I hemmed and hawed and ended up saying I had to run, my phone wasn't working, and I'd get back to her.

Cornered criminals can make circumstances harder on themselves. In a frantic attempt to provide a coherent clinical scenario, I tried to cover my actions by making a fictitious medical chart for Ruth, ex post facto. The dates on most of the prescriptions were for after she had left the country, so this chart didn't make any sense. Later, it was one more incriminating thing to explain to the medical board.

This pharmacist should have called *America's Dumbest Criminals*. Instead, she called the police. Several weeks later, in February 2005, the other shoe dropped, in the form of Bruno and Rufus visiting my office.

The family weekend rushed by, and soon it was once again time to say good-bye and to head back to Tannenberg. I had been dreading this moment. This second leave-taking was harder. "Why do you have to go away *again*? It's not fair." The kids were hysterical. I knew that I had only two weeks left, but to a six-year-old and a five-year-old, this is equivalent to forever. Rehab was starting to feel like prison. Enough is enough.

Immediately on my return to Tannenberg, Nate hit me up for a drug test, personally supervising. "Good to the last drop, Grinspoon. I hope for your sake you didn't screw this up."

Tannenberg seemed the same as when I had left seventy-two hours earlier, save for a couple of relapses, which were hot on the gossip circle. One nurse made a spectacular return from her home visit by falling out of her car, dead drunk and grinning like the cat that swallowed the goldfish. She drunkenly told everyone that she loved them, especially the irate Tannenberg staff, trying to hug them out of absolute love as they screamed at her. Later, she explained that this relapse caught her as much by surprise as everyone else. She described her pit stop at the liquor store as "sleepwalking" and couldn't remember the drive back to Tannenberg.

Despite the external sameness, my relationship to the reality of being at Tannenberg had been transformed by spending time at home with my kids. My inner clock was ticking loudly, and I couldn't wait to be finished. I had no patience left for the same inane lectures and the endless talk about God curing our addictions.

To pass the time, I baited the locals. "Now, why would God go to the trouble of creating a disease, if only to then cure it? Is he bored? If we can't see God, how do we really know he's there listening?" One of the local carpenters channeled his inner Kierkegaard and answered, in an angry southern accent, "I can't

see electricity but I know it's there when I turn on a light switch."
Touché. The room erupted into applause at my expense.

My post-rehab Scylla (felony criminal charges) and Charybdis
(the medical board) were starting to loom larger, as it was now a
matter of weeks not months before I had to deal with them. They
were transitioning from hypothetical to real, and I couldn't stand
having them hanging over my head. I was chomping at the bit to
either beat the rap or to bend over and begin my punishment.

My older brother, David, was approved to visit me, contingent
on a negative drug test after my home visit. Tall and charming,
with frizzy hair and a soul patch, David is a writer of awesome
Carl Sagan–like books, a musician, and an astrobiologist who
specializes in life on other planets and the effect humans have on
Earth. I have always looked up to him, and I was delighted that
he would be landing on Planet Tannenberg to help me understand the life forms here.

David and I had wandered around rural Zimbabwe together for
six weeks in 1989, time and again barely escaping with our hides,
dodging beatings, the elements, political violence, predatory animals, and starvation. It didn't help that we were sometimes more
stoned than the dictates of safety might have recommended.
Since then, we have shared a close and special bond.

Once, we managed to get locked in the Great Zimbabwe ruins
after dark, where there was no limit of humans or animals that
would have savored making a meal of us. We had the address
of a friend of a friend's house, and we ended up banging on the
barbed-wire fence at the back of their compound, and pleading to
be rescued from our fate.

Over the snarling of their attack dogs, we shouted, "Hello
there, we are friends of the Joneses who are friends of the Smiths,
and we are visiting Zimbabwe and, foolishly, we somehow seem
to be locked in here after dark, and we really don't want to be
eaten alive. Is there any way you could allow us in for the night?"
They eventually allowed us in, once they convinced themselves
that we weren't marauding bandits or con artists.

Now, our zany adventures were to continue, for one glorious
weekend, in the sober world of rehab, in East Bumfuck, North

Carolina. David stoically attended the AA meetings with me, which, in retrospect, was iffy, because you aren't supposed to attend if you aren't yourself an alcoholic or an addict. His first wife had struggled with drinking, so it wasn't entirely alien to him.

David found the Southern Baptist AA experience interesting in a cultural sense, while, at that point in my rehab career, I was so bored with it that I was willing to pull my own teeth out, or set myself on fire, to make it more interesting.

One of the meetings David attended was about gratitude. I initially found this to be an important and positive message, but it lost its significance after about two hundred thousand repetitions. It's healthier to be appreciative of what we have than to focus on what's wrong in our lives. I get it. But I'd be most grateful to stop hearing about how I should be feeling grateful all the time.

At that particular meeting, I was sincerely grateful to have a fellow atheist and skeptic to witness this mumbo-jumbo cultist crap I was tired of being force-fed. David, who found the discussion touching, was also obliged to admit that these meetings were "pretty silly" when assessed solely on their content. It wasn't easy being a secular humanist surrounded by religious people, or by people overly enmeshed in the insular culture of AA.

Our reward for surviving these meetings was mini golf. I didn't inflict Hooters on David.

Experiencing even these few days of life at Tannenberg with David, who is so deeply anchored in my past, helped bridge my two worlds. It gave my experiences at Tannenberg a sense of reality and context, which had been sorely lacking. Thanks for the reality, David!

On departing, David said, "It's really cool that you're here, getting better. I know that, at times, it seems like a lot of unscientific God crap to you, but I'm really proud of what you're doing, and I'm happy to have you healthy again." I responded, "God and the universe are one!" This is an inside joke, referring to a young Baha'i named Derek, who had followed David and me around for the whole six weeks that we traveled across Zimbabwe together.

Derek repeated this saying over and over again. David and I said this to each other whenever we wanted to communicate how important our connection to each other is.

On my last day at Tannenberg, there was a short graduation ceremony where we sat around in a circle and passed a coin along, which I was to keep. Each member of the recovery community wished me sobriety and health, as they rubbed the germs from their hands into this coin. Lyle had already physically left, and I had already mentally left, so the ceremony felt somewhat pro forma.

When it came time to say my good-byes to my roommates, Rudy came up to me and, to my utter shock and surprise, paid me back forty dollars he owed me. I would have sooner predicted that he grew wings, feathers, and a beak, and flew off into the sunset. "Peter, you've been a good friend to me. I haven't had many friends. I'd like to keep in touch. Here's my number."

This posed a quandary. If someone is drowning, how can you refuse to take their hand? Is it possible that I had unknowingly activated a kernel of goodness in Rudy? Or was he going to find me in Boston and plop down on my sofa, chain-smoke, and rifle through my spare change? The thought of him and my kids in the same room was too discordant and scary so, with great flourish, I wrote down a fake phone number for him to never reach me at. I do hope that he stays sober, and that he finds a less antagonistic way to connect to people.

It was time to pack up the car and head back to Boston. As much as I had hated the idea of rehab, and had resisted it with every molecule of my body, I was quite emotional upon packing up to leave. I knew that I'd keep in touch with Lyle, but I also knew that most of these people, who were the heart and soul of my recovery, were people I'd never see again.

I also worried about whether I had truly recovered, and whether I was going to be all right once the intensive scrutiny of rehab was over. I am such a bullshit artist, I was worried that I had convinced myself, as much as everyone else, that I was in recovery, but that the same addictive insanity was going to come roaring back.

As a final bad omen, as I was backing out of the parking lot, the finance director of Tannenberg sideswiped my car. "I'm sorry, sweetheart, I wasn't paying attention and was just gabbing on my cell phone." As long as my car would still physically move forward, I was heading back to Boston.

As I drove back to Boston after my "extreme makeover," looking back and trying to make sense of my behavior, there seems to be a disconnect between two distinct aspects of Peter Grinspoon that had coexisted in the same body. One Peter was externally perceived to be hardworking, full of idealism, humor, compassion, and a genuine desire to help people: the medical student who was a "star," the resident who was a "gem," generous, and open-minded. My grandmother, the ultimate authority on all things, maintained that I was a "mensch." Doctors, staff, families, and patients all liked me and appreciated my ability to communicate and to empathize.

Operating independently, within the same body, was the Peter who skulked in the shadows and stole pills, who wrote fake prescriptions, formed criminal allegiances with patients, and manipulated his colleagues into prescribing Vicodin for him. This version of Peter was emotionally AWOL from his marriage, and lived in an increasingly isolated, surrealistic dreamworld of pills and deception.

It wasn't just H. who had been concerned. After one New Year's Eve celebration, when I got overly wasted to the point of being incoherent and blacking out, H.'s best friend revoked our status as alternate guardians for their kids. This stung. On another night, my dad saw me sway when we were leaving his house after a dinner together. He asked me if there was anything to what H. was saying about my drug use. "Of course not. She's paranoid."

We had a tense family meeting with my parents and my in-laws, all of whom were invested in trying to save our faltering marriage. I promised to get my act together, and H. promised to be less haranguing and punishing. Neither of us was able to keep our promise.

Friends and relatives must have eventually noticed that wherever I visited, pills would go missing, and that I was always rustling around the upstairs of their homes. Several cousins said they were worried about me. My favorite cousin, one of my favorite people on the planet, said, "I love you but I don't trust you." These words cut to the core.

My primary care doc angrily warned me, "Don't ever again call me at home," after I called him on a Saturday evening looking for Vicodin. I had milked "professional courtesy" one too many times.

Even my twin brother, the last person on earth to doubt me, voiced concern. He said, "You were stoned out of your mind on the day that you and H. moved into your new house. Why would you get that high? It was like you weren't even here."

To me, the real mystery is how I was able to live with myself. If I saw anyone else succumbing to this, I'd rush to get them help, corner them, coerce them, browbeat them, threaten them, coordinate an intervention, do anything it took to get them into treatment. Why was I so oblivious about it in my own life?

Part of the answer is that addiction makes you fundamentally selfish. At the time, I didn't feel particularly guilty about any of the awful things I was doing. They say that an addict will steal your wallet and then spend hours helping you look for it.

The only thing that penetrated the barriers and haze of my addicted mind, like in *Horton Hears a Who!*, was the voice of my kids, asking for a dad who was present and who loved them. On some level, I knew that I was letting Annie and Milo down, and this made me feel rotten inside. But these sentiments are little match for a full-blown addiction. I know a doc who taped a small picture of his young kids to a pill bottle to dissuade himself from taking the pills. It didn't work, and only served to make him feel guiltier.

There's a notion that the craziest things a drug addict does are when he or she is high. This may be true in cases of extreme intoxication, like when our childhood friend Will dropped acid and tried to kill Martin's college girlfriend. In medical school, we heard and saw pictures about a case where a guy who was high on coke ran straight through a glass door.

In my experience, with a hindsight view of the wreckage, when I was on the drugs I mostly vegged out and kept to myself, but almost all of my dishonest, criminal, and insane behavior occurred when I was in withdrawal, desperate to procure my next fix.

I ordered my whole world around this pursuit, which involved an astounding amount of manipulation. It was like being possessed by an alien impulse. My "drug radar" was always on, continually emitting a low-frequency beacon for opportunities to score. I would befriend neighbors or create social situations primarily in order to replenish my supplies.

Upon entering the house of an acquaintance, I'd feel my pulse quickening as my sense of craving escalated. I'd bide my time, participate in the dinner or brunch conversation, and wait for my opportunity to steal upstairs and begin hunting and gathering. The perfect pretext was my beeper going off and the need for a private phone conversation.

When free, I immediately started rustling through medicine cabinets, rifling through drawers, pocketing whatever pills I found. I tore off and flushed away any identifying information from pill bottles. I put a piece of tissue in the pill bottles so the pills wouldn't rattle in my pocket when I came back down to rejoin the company.

My ears strained for the sound of footsteps, and, on occasion, I came close to being caught and had to ad lib. "I was answering a page, and then I saw your bookshelf and started looking at the books," or "I was looking for a place where my cell phone has clear reception."

Open houses were outstanding places to score, and it just so happened that one of H.'s passions was house hunting, in search of the perfect suburban fortress. The bathroom off the master bedroom was the most fruitful place to search, though the night-stands weren't bad. People would often hide their prescriptions in the top drawer of their dresser, among their clean socks and underwear. I was monomaniacal.

H. once walked in on me as I was pocketing a bottle of codeine in a master bedroom and threatened to call the police. I mollified her by putting the pills back while she watched. I managed to squirrel them away again before we left. She went up to check, but I had put Tylenol in the bottle so that it looked full, and had hidden the pills under the spare tire of my car. These scenes repeated themselves over and over again.

But none of this compared to the line I crossed with Cindy, and four other patients I shared prescriptions with. Even though it was a different type of prescription violation that invited Bruno and Rufus into my office, I think that this boundary violation with patients and pills is what was most troubling to my conscience. It was also potentially lethal to my medical career, and nearly impossible to explain to the medical board in a way that made it sound like I should be practicing medicine.

As my behavior was degenerating, and I was facing a growing chorus of concerned family/friends/colleagues/therapists, I tried on many occasions to quit. Every single time I was dope sick, wracked with flu-like symptoms and depression, I swore off the pills permanently. It wasn't lost to me how frequently this pattern was recurring. There's only so much suffering any person can ignore.

There were countless times when I forced myself to flush bottles of pills down the toilet, to prevent myself from taking them. Anything short of flushing was futile, because I would find a way to retrieve them, like a newly quit smoker trying to salvage a crumpled pack of cigarettes from the garbage.

Oftentimes, as I watched the pills swirl down the drain, I would see them, if for just a moment, for the poison that they are. Once they were gone, I usually felt a sharp pang of remorse for flushing them. It felt like some of my little buddies had been washed away, friends I had gone to great trouble, risk, or expense to procure.

My newfound sobriety might last a week or so, if I didn't stumble upon anything, until I'd find myself driving to CVS, pulled along by the gravitational force of the pills restlessly waiting for me in small bottles behind the pharmacy counter. During these excursions, I was conscious, but also in a trance or a dissociative state, like the Manchurian candidate, with an inner directive that circumvents the other brain waves. The small area in my brain that craves drugs, my reward center, which is less than a cubic centimeter in size, overpowered the rest of my brain and had utter control over my actions and intentions.

Whenever I walked toward the back of CVS, to the prescription area, my vision would change, heighten, and focus, and the labels on the bottles of narcotics would glow neon and seem to float, dance, hover, and beckon, as I was handing the prescription to the pharmacist. Acting as casually as I could, I paced the aisles while my prescription was being filled, and flipped through magazines like Us, written for vapid people who live in a world of suspended disbelief.

As I was waiting, my mind swirled with what-ifs. What if they don't accept the prescription? What if it's too soon to refill? What if the pharmacist gets suspicious? Why is this taking them so long? I was usually getting sicker by the minute.

Once my name was called, I paid, and they handed me the small orange pill bottle labeled VICODIN, packaged neatly in a white paper bag that was folded over and stapled. It was all I could do not to sprint out of the pharmacy, bumping into people in my zeal to be outside. I was sweating and shaking, a Pavlovian response to the burst of pleasure, and the relief of discomfort, I was about to experience.

Finally outside of CVS, standing in the vestibule by the automatic doors, I would swallow six to eight pills, blithely ignoring the catastrophic impression this might have made on a colleague or a patient, if they had happened to walk into the pharmacy just then. Like a dog worrying a bone, I'd be seen struggling to rip or chew off the labels on the pill bottles, to evade detection by H.

Now, as I was driving home to Boston, fortified with ninety

days of treatment, I could only hope that I would be able to do better.

What tools was I given to help fend off my addiction? What higher power was going to bring out the best in me? Physically, I was the same as I had been three months earlier, when I had driven down, except for the chemical adjustments that my treatment team had made, with some drugs stopped and others started. So what mental or psychic change was I harboring that was going to help me to confront the wreckage of my former life, and to avoid the same temptations that had so recently torpedoed my career?

Being away at a residential treatment program was an awesome, unique opportunity to view my life with some critical distance, and to work with a therapist such as Nate, to help reevaluate what is, at core, most important to me. Life doesn't offer these opportunities very often. As Lyle once said, rehab is "an awesome experience; too bad you have to be a drunk or a druggie to do it."

For many people, the "higher power" that unifies and animates their recovery is ready-made for them. Their higher power is the same god that they have always believed in, whom they now enlist to help with their addiction. Their god, who already exists, has to pay more attention to a problem that they have now developed.

Gandhi viewed all religions as the same, and I think this can be said about people's higher powers as well. What differs is the language they use to describe and conceptualize their higher power. What is common to all of us is that our higher power elevates our souls enough to transcend our addictions.

In my case, I had to beg, borrow, and steal in order to cobble together my higher power. I needed to imbue it with enough force and meaning to lift me out of the hopeless morass I was mired in.

My higher power can best be described as a rugged idealism that sprouts up no matter how much my life is falling apart. This idealism was formed in the crucible of my ultra-academic background, in response to my brother Danny's death. It was nurtured by the Famous Astronomers of the world, and it was confirmed and strengthened by my experience of Greenpeace and of people linked together trying to improve the world.

This idealism has always been present within me. It was alongside me in the frozen wastelands of Chernobyl. It was there in the room with me when we were telling the submerged six-year-old's family that he had frozen in the lake. I see this idealism in my children's eyes, no matter how much H. and I are fighting.

But it was lost to me during my addiction, and needed to be reclaimed, dusted off, recharged, and embraced. It was my only hope.

PART THREE

Reentry

Having just finished my stint in rehab at Tannenberg Rehab, in July of 2005 I drove my dinged-up and pollen-covered car back to Boston in a mingled state of near-euphoria, optimism, and fear. In drastic contrast to my voyage down, ninety days earlier, the molecules of my foot now sought out the gas pedal, not the brake.

I had survived rehab, which I was originally so dubious about, with my sense of self intact. As far as I could tell, I hadn't been brainwashed or reprogrammed or forced to join any cult. In fact, quite the opposite. I didn't want anything more to do with AA for the next thousand lifetimes.

I was convinced that my "degree" in rehab would render null and void the criminal charges that were still hanging over my head. Once the authorities understood that addiction is a brain disease, which was not entirely under my control or my fault, they would work with me collaboratively to move forward.

These criminal charges pertained to the addict I used to be, not the new and improved Peter. It wasn't me who committed these crimes. I was innocent because it was the old me, not the new me, it was the addicted part of my brain, who committed these prescription violations. It was the disease itself acting out.

As far as I was concerned, my case was already closed. I couldn't wait to explain this to the judge, who probably needed some education around addiction for good measure. I was happy to provide it in the form of a concise, doctorly lecture.

"Your Honor, I know that you, like most judges, are a conventional thinker, and have very old-fashioned conceptions about addiction. I'm here to educate you, so please pay attention. Addiction is not a moral failing, as you have been led to believe, but a chemical brain disease that requires leniency, understanding, and treatment, not punishment. Let my people go!"

I wouldn't be surprised if the judge even apologized for allowing the criminal charges in the first place. "Doctor, this was a misunderstanding. We didn't understand that you had a *brain disease*. None of this is your fault. We are so sorry for wasting your time, and we will be glad to reimburse your legal fees."

Along the same lines, I thought my rehab degree would mollify the medical board. Quid pro quo. I'd paid my dues, now they should step out of the way and let me get back to work. It was the old Peter, not the current version, who wrote fake scrips, shared prescriptions with patients, and stole drugs. Distant past. Ancient history. No use crying over spilled milk.

I'd been out of work for more than three months, and was more than ready to pick up where I left off, if these ignorant old farts would only let me. Solomon must be wrong. The board wouldn't make me wait a year for something that wasn't my fault. It sounded like they could use a vigorous lecture on addiction too.

"Assembled members of the medical board, I have to say it's somewhat disappointing that you, as physicians, don't know anything about addiction, and are still living in the Dark Ages, where addicts are mindlessly punished, instead of treated..."

My irrational exuberance stemmed from having just spent ninety days immersed in a community of people who accepted my addiction as a medical condition that can be treated and put into remission.

Many, but by no means all, of the people in my life somehow managed to still love and like me, despite my having lied to them and stolen their medications. The phone calls with friends and cousins, aunts and colleagues, placed from the extremely public phone wall at Tannenberg, kept me in touch not only with the outside world but with an important part of myself that needed to remain intact. I needed to feel that I was still worth forgiving.

If I weren't so blissed out from my rehab experience, floating on the "pink cloud" of new recovery, I might not have been in such blithe denial about the challenges awaiting me in Boston: an explosively disintegrating marriage, felony criminal charges that possibly could involve jail time, a medical board with a lynch-mob mentality that wanted to atomize my license to practice, and two children whose lives were imploding around them even more rapidly than mine was.

The "take home" from Tannenberg is that addiction is a treatable disease that I wasn't entirely responsible for, due to my brain chemistry. At the expense of $40K, and ninety profoundly long days, I thought that I had earned my "get out of jail free" card.

As I was soon to learn the hard way, most people, who aren't living in the sheltered, insular world of recovery, don't feel this way. In the real world, crimes are punished, without nuance or second thought. Examples are made of people who don't do what they are supposed to.

Even worse, despite my rehab degree and despite my being enveloped in the language and spirit of recovery, the embers of my addiction were still faintly glowing underneath this soggy mud fortress of recovery, waiting for a gust of wind and some dry sticks.

As I voyaged back to Boston, H. and I discussed which home port would welcome me and my dusty and dented Subaru. Ninety days earlier, when I left for North Carolina, I was staying with my parents at my childhood home in Wellesley, having been kicked out by H., with screamed threats of not seeing the children, divorce, poverty, restraining orders, retribution, calling the police, and with my possessions scattered on the front lawn.

"Peter, I think that we did well during your home visit a few weeks ago. Do you want to try coming home directly from Tannenberg, and we can give things another chance?" I missed my kids and my home; there's no way I could resist this invitation from H. back to our family home in Hyde Park.

All four of us nurtured the fantasy that this honeymoon would continue, that our marital problems would follow my addiction into the vapors of recovery, and that we could once again be a united family. I kept hearing Nate's voice in my head: "Go back clean 'n sober, see what happens. There's yer test. There's yer answer."

It was destroying me not to be living with the kids, and this influenced my decision to return to the marriage. I was wracked with guilt about having already caused so much dislocation to their childhood.

I was having a great deal of trouble forgiving myself for the times I nodded off when caring for them, or the times I was ill-tempered from withdrawal, rushing to finish reading their stories, hurrying to put them to bed so that I could go zone out, smoke pot, pop some pills, go back to my office. The only recourse to being overwhelmed with guilt was to follow Nate's advice: "Just do the next right thing and all this stuff will work out... You'll feel better. Things fall back into place."

Regardless of my issues, or H.'s contribution to our marital problems, we had brought Annie and Milo into the world. They didn't choose their parents, or to be born in the first place. They deserved a shot at a secure childhood, with swim lessons, play-dates, soccer games, birthday parties, sleepovers, adventures, and trips to the toy store. They deserved to grow up without having to experience their parents screaming at each other, their dad zoned out, or their mom screeching and smashing things. This wasn't supposed to be *The Liars' Club* or *Angela's Ashes*. There were enough sad stories out there.

Upon my return to the marital home, the kids couldn't have been happier to have both parents together, like sheepdog puppies no longer anxious that the herd is scattered. No more broken, stuttering phone calls from rehab, "I love you, I miss you too." Click. No more missing me or crying themselves to sleep.

H. was warm and welcoming, though, given the intensity of the rancor that had passed between us a mere three months before, we were both leery. Gone with the screaming was the easy and comfortable familiarity. We were polite and awkward together.

The physical structure of my home was exactly as I had left it, with its Victorian decor and its sedimentary layer of plastic toys covering the floor. Its very familiarity depressed me, reminding me of the hell I had recently been through, what all four of us had been through, the fights between H. and me, and the seemingly insurmountable obstacles I had to confront. My first instinct was to sneak up to the back porch and take a toke, or to get back in my car and drive away.

Inwardly, I was reeling from all of the changes I had been through, as if in ninety days I had shed lifetimes, and skins. I felt constrained, as if I were walking on eggshells, not wanting to upset a delicate new world order. Nate had warned me, "You've changed, they haven't; it's hard going home."

The eagerness and hope I saw shining in the faces of my children unsettled me because I had no guarantee that my marriage to H. was going to succeed, that the fights and separations wouldn't start up again. The absolute last thing I wanted was to dash the hopes they were nurturing, to retraumatize them, if H. and I were to melt down again.

Grasping at the straws of their hope, which I saw reflected in their faces, I suspended disbelief, and managed to ignore the gathering storm clouds swirling around H. and me.

My first full day in Boston featured a return to Solomon's office. After a somber ride up the elevator to the fourteenth floor, I had a long wait in the lobby. I tried to block out the high-pitched chatter of the secretaries, which was so carefree and bland, in contrast to the seriousness of my situation, so that I could concentrate on finishing *Humboldt's Gift*, which, prose like a drug, removed me from my problems.

Solomon finally entered, and led me back to his office.

"Solomon, with all this, I succeeded in rehab. That has to help, a lot. Were you joking when you said I might have to wait a year? Where do we stand?"

"Peter, we are now still in purgatory."

"What?? I've been working my ass off for ninety days. That has to help."

The twelve steps of Alcoholics Anonymous liberally reference God and a higher power, but they don't make any mention of purgatory. I asked for clarification.

According to Solomon, "Your rehab degree will help if you don't screw up again. It's still going to be a long path, and neither the judge nor the medical board trust you at all right now. The criminal charges are first; they potentially have the most serious consequences. But the board is going to have a problem with this other stuff," meaning my boundary violations, including sharing prescriptions with patients.

Post-rehab, I was envisioning a rapid return to work, and I didn't have the most realistic notions of when that might be. Solomon said, "It will be at least twelve to eighteen months before they will even consider having you back, and that is only if everything goes perfectly." Eighteen months? Are you joking? What am I supposed to do with myself? I was used to dodging the authorities and getting slaps on the wrist. This was a full-body bitch slap.

Solomon and I discussed how much to disclose voluntarily to the medical board during my looming interrogation. This was not a straightforward issue. No one discloses everything. The board knows that.

The more I voluntarily admitted to, the more trouble I would get in, and the longer it would be until I would be allowed to return to work. This makes it tempting to hold back incriminating details.

However, if the board uncovered anything significant that I didn't disclose, I would be up shit's creek. That's how people get their license revoked for five years, not just suspended for a year or two.

I know someone from a recovery meeting who told the board that she had just started using cocaine, to make it look like she had had a recent, innocent lapse of judgment, rather than an addiction that spanned years. When the board received a discharge summary from her rehab program explaining that she had used cocaine frequently in high school and in college, they unceremoniously told her to find another profession, in the form of a license revocation.

Part of me wanted to just tell everyone everything, to get it off my chest. Then there would be no surprises later. I told Solomon that being open and honest was consistent with my recovery. Solomon couldn't ethically counsel me to withhold information, but he cautioned me to be prudent: "You want to be honest, but not stupid."

This reminded me of the discussion we doctors had at rehab, about how "honesty" is saying you have an addiction and you did things you regret, whereas "truthfulness" is incriminating yourself by telling them about each of your criminal violations.

Moving on to the criminal charges, Solomon explained that "it wasn't impossible" that I would go to jail, depending on the judge, but that it was unlikely because, even though it is a felony, it was nonviolent, and I am a "first offender, without a record." (Thank God none of the criminal charges from Greenpeace had stuck around…) Solomon then told me that he had had a "fairly good" conversation with the assistant district attorney (the prosecuting attorney). Two more likely possibilities were being considered: pretrial probation or a continuation without a finding (CWOF).

Solomon explained that pretrial probation, the best possible outcome, meant satisfying all of the requirements of a probation officer for several years. If I was able to jump through whatever additional hoops the probation officer required, the criminal charges would expire after a certain date.

More ominously, a CWOF, pronounced "quaff," is the legal equivalent of the Twilight Zone. While it doesn't require an admission of guilt, it would stay on my criminal record forever, and could factor into any legal problems I had in the future.

A CWOF would make a return to medicine logistically impossible, because Medicare considers a CWOF equivalent to a guilty plea. If it is related to a prescription violation, Medicare gives an automatic five-year suspension. It is impossible to practice primary care without being credentialed through Medicare.

I have colleagues who have finished their SHP contract and are green-lighted by the medical board to return, but who still can't practice medicine, years later, because of this unintended consequence of a CWOF, which prohibits their participation in Medicare.

According to Solomon, "We'll just put our best foot forward and hope to avoid the CWOF."

Solomon then told me that they were trying to contact Rufus, from the state police, to see if he would go along with the pretrial probation. Rufus?? He was the calorically challenged officer who had overzealously crushed my finger into the computer screen while taking my fingerprints. Since when does Rufus's opinion matter? He's not the judge; he's just a policeman who happened to be assigned to my case. I thought I was done with Rufus. The eternal recurrence was recurring.

When I last saw him, Rufus had been visibly salivating at the chance of convicting a doctor. It was something to tell his grandkids about. He wasn't going to agree to anything less than death by hanging. The district attorney set my court date for a few weeks later.

Solomon advised me to get to SHP as soon as possible, to start drug screens right away, so there would be continuity from my tests at rehab. "No matter what, do not flunk a drug screen."

The next day, at the Taj Mahal/Medical Society of Massachusetts in Waltham, the director of SHP saw me reading *The Caine Mutiny* while I waited to sign my new three-year contract with them. He told me I had good taste in books, and said that he remembered the movie. I told him that I felt like I was going down with the ship, along with Captain Queeg. He looked alarmed. (Much later, when I was sleep-deprived from training an uncooperative puppy, I accidentally referred to this book, while recommending it to Martin, as *The Canine Mutiny*.)

The staff at SHP were encouraged by the positive report they received from Tannenberg, and they quoted statistics to me that gave me, as a doctor, around an 80 to 90 percent chance of success, if I passed my drug tests and fulfilled the other parts of my contract, which included attending physician support groups and meeting with my addiction therapist, Ben, weekly, as well as with my SHP mentor, Dr. Stern, every month.

Under my polite demeanor, despite genuine respect for the

good people of SHP who were trying to help me, my attitude was best described as "fuck you very much." This "contract" was not voluntary, but compulsory if I ever wanted to practice medicine again. It felt extremely restrictive and degrading. I thought that I had this under control, and didn't need to dance like a trained pony.

I was anxious about passing my first drug screen, scheduled for the next day, because, on my drive home from Tannenberg, in an act of defiance for all the hours upon hours of listening to people talk about God and forgiveness, about humility and becoming a better person, I drank a margarita with my medical school room-mate, Stavros, whom I visited in Baltimore.

I don't even like alcohol. As Thomas De Quincey said, "I do not readily believe that any man having once tasted the divine luxuries of opium will afterwards descend to the gross and mor-tal enjoyments of alcohol." Amen, brother. As Nate would say, I was being a "rebel without a clue." Now I was hoping that this one syrupy margarita wouldn't undo me.

SHP required that I meet with Ben right away. Unfortunately, Ben's office was located in the Faulkner Hospital where, less than four months earlier, I had been employed as a primary care doc-tor. Despite trying to convince myself that addiction is a treatable disease, not my fault, etc., I was mortified to walk into my hospi-tal. I discussed this with Ben over the phone.

> "Peter, your shame comes from a neurotic and unreal fear that others will reject you."
> "Ben, I just left four doctors and thousands of patients in the lurch. When they see me, an angry mob is going to spon-taneously take form. I am going to be tarred and feath-ered. Or tarred and bandaged. I'm not sure where you are getting the 'neurotic and unreal' part of this. Did they teach you that in therapy school?"
> "You are saying this because you are acting out. This is your addiction talking. You need to stay calm and trust the process."

"That is so easy for you to say! You have a job. By the way, have you quit smoking yet? Did I mention that it's hypocritical for an addiction counselor to smoke?"

"This is your therapy, not mine, so shut up about the smoking for now."

As I spun through the revolving door at the front entrance to the hospital, I kept my eyes trained on the ground and gave my former office a wide berth, hoping not to bump into anyone I had ever met, or who had ever even heard about me. I immediately almost crashed into a cluster of my patients on my way to Ben's office. They were likely discussing the juicy gossip of their doctor who had disappeared from practice.

Several gathered around me at once, waiting expectantly for an explanation as to why I was not currently performing my obligations as their doctor. Unable to fly or become invisible, I claimed poor health. Unfortunately, I looked in the prime of life, and I didn't have a limp, a scar, an amputation, an attached IV, a dangling catheter bag, or anything that would add credibility to this explanation. I thought that, for the next appointment with Ben, I should either maim myself or at least shave my head so that my patients would assume I had cancer.

Farther down the hallway, I bumped into a friendly but supercilious cardiologist who asked me point-blank, "Do you still work here?" I answered, "I'm not sure." What I meant was "I've been terminated, but I'm not sure I believe all of this is really happening." Inside, I burned with shame.

I still held on to the romantic notion that, even though the hospital had terminated me, my medical practice would one day offer me my job back, based on what a friendly and perceptive primary care doctor I was. I had no logical grounds for optimism. The letter they sent to my patients, explaining that I was no longer part of the practice, sounded pretty definitive and permanent. It may as well have said that I was one of the pioneers gone on a one-way ticket to colonize Mars.

When I finally made it to his office, Ben was as supportive to me as he could be, under the circumstances. His voice was raspy from chain-smoking. "Peter, keep your head up. This sucks, but you've got to keep the faith. Remember, it is what it is." I started grappling with this non sequitur, which he employs at least a dozen times during a typical therapy session.

"Please stop saying 'It is what it is.' I studied this in philosophy. That is a tautological argument. Or circular reasoning: *a* equals *a*. It is what it is. Quit smoking yet? Let me guess: It still is what it is."

As Ben was gasping for air, he said, "Don't mind about me. How are you doing with all this? I told you that you wouldn't bump into any patients."

"They *surrounded* me. It was like a medieval execution. Ben, you should try a twelve-step program for tobacco. Tobacco Anonymous is supposed to be quite effective."

"Think of what you've already accomplished: You are still alive, you are in recovery, you are earning back trust, and you are sorting out the rest of your life."

"You make it sound so good, and so noble, but I keep getting bad news. And things with H. are getting worse."

During this hectic time of preparing to defend criminal charges in court, I was hoping that on the home front things would be quiet, so that I could reconnect with the kids, regroup, and focus my energies on my upcoming trial. I didn't have the internal or external resources to fight a two-front war.

Within a few months of returning from rehab, I started to cheat, or, in drug slang, I started "chipping." A few pills here and there. I was drug-tested every week, and I knew that a positive test would be reported to the medical board. The board didn't need any more ammunition in order to crucify me.

These sporadic pills caused me far more anxiety than they were worth. I lived in a constant state of fear. Occasionally, SHP would order a second test during a given week, to keep us honest. This testing schedule translated into a slightly higher than 20 percent chance I'd get called in for a drug test on any given day, Monday through Friday. There were no tests on the weekends.

If I didn't get called by eight a.m. on a Friday, or if there had already been a second test that week, say on Tuesday or Wednesday, I knew that there wouldn't be a test until Monday. I was allowed to take my test as late as 4:00 p.m. on Monday afternoons. This left about eighty hours between Friday mornings and Monday afternoons.

Most drugs are detectable in the urine for no more than seventy-two hours. Even if I had the worst luck, and was called on Monday for a test, which would occur only one-fifth of the time, I probably would pass my drug screen on Monday if I used on Friday.

After taking pills on Friday afternoons, I would wait with panic the next few weeks for my drug tests to return. I would drink loads of water and work out in the gym for hours, in the desperate belief that this would help me metabolize the drugs faster. I drank so much water on the morning of the tests, I got in trouble with SHP for too many dilute tests. Dr. Stern, who is nobody's fool, said, "Be very careful with your water intake. We are concerned that you might be hiding something."

On Wednesday, August 24, 2005, six weeks after returning from rehab, I mapped the days back in my diary, counting back to the Saturday when I took pills, to reassure myself that I would pass the test: "1–3 days limit, was 4 days with dilution, and with 1 time use (therefore no buildup) meant to catch daily use not sporadic or to catch use of long half-life." I then gave myself a motivational speech: "big picture, kids, exercise, read, write, things good with H., will work again, enthusiasm, energy, motivation, it's just crazy and suicidal what you are doing, don't be cute, Cut It Out, this disease will Bury you."

Both H. and I remained hopeful that we could start a new chapter, in spite of our period of ugliness right before I left for rehab. She would need to forgive and forget countless episodes of bad behavior on my part. And there was one memory from before, that most powerfully haunted my own hopes for the future. One evening, I had been startled out of my bedroom by the intermittent sound of breaking glass. The sound was coming from the floor just below me. Home intruder? Rock through the window via juvenile delinquent? Vengeful patient? Anti-Semitic hordes?

As I rushed down the stairs, hearing the children's concerned cries as they awakened from their sleep, there was another loud crash, which led me to the kitchen, where H. was collapsed on the kitchen floor, sobbing, in a heap of jagged detritus. She had just swept the contents of the shelves in the fridge onto the floor, and she had just smashed several plates against the wall.

When she noticed my presence, she turned on me, pointed expansively at the wreckage, and screamed, "You bastard, this is all your fault!" (For marrying her? For not using a condom? For buying plates? For owning a kitchen?) She then heaved another plate against the wall, which seemed to shatter in slow motion.

Despite both of our best efforts, I was never to enjoy a positive new beginning with H. She had made it clear from the outset that my new role as "house husband" was not to be venerated, or even respected, in our household. Nor was it to be lauded as a modern and progressive reversal of gender roles. There would be no celebration of a dad spending extra time with the kids, no time to read or relax. No naps. No sexual favors. No downtime. No nights out with my own friends. No lounging on the front porch over coffee.

Until I started working again and was bringing in a salary, I was in the doghouse, and I was going to pay for what I had done. Her philosophy of doghouse was that it should be maximum security, with major disincentives. She threatened to force me to work at Home Depot, so that I wouldn't continue to be a "useless husband." Orange (Home Depot apron) is the new black.

An immediate problem was that H. didn't trust me at all. She had always been on the profoundly controlling side, but now she seized control of the utilities, shut down the media, dismissed the judiciary, and closely supervised my every movement. She practically expected me to check in with her before going to the bathroom.

In the context of my new, lessened stature, she felt unrestrained in ordering me around: "Drive with two hands," "Make the bed," and "Come to the door when I call you." Or, "This house was spotless when you arrived back from rehab." When I complained, she replied, "You are not allowed to speak" and "Your point of view doesn't count," followed by a slammed door. I sensed she was angry.

H. continued her postmarital habit of talking in her sleep. Her nightly unconscious angry monologues became far more vitriolic than previously. It's hard to fall asleep to a muttered "You ass-hole, no-good drug addict."

Even when I could fall asleep, H. developed a new habit of waking me up in the middle of the night, out of a sound sleep, often several times in one night. "The water's running," "Can you check the heater?" and "Can you get a flashlight?" In the morning she either didn't remember or wouldn't admit to these intrusions. I believe that when she woke up in the night, she just couldn't stand to see me peacefully sleeping, given what I had done to our lives.

By my fifth day back home, I was feeling the possibility of ten-der intimacy, which H. and I both craved, slipping away from us. I tried to convince myself that things were still going to work out for the best, writing in my diary, "H. is kind of irritable but she's still loving and nice."

The next three weeks passed quickly, in a blur of recovery meet-ings, drug tests, therapy sessions with Ben, household chores and childcare, sleep-fragmented nights, and slowly escalating tension with H. I doggedly submerged into the roiling waters of my sub-conscious any thoughts about the criminal charges I was about to face. Until it was time to go to court.

Accompanied again by Solomon's understudy, Eric, I again climbed the steps of the West Roxbury Municipal Courthouse, went through the vintage metal detectors and the detailed pat-down by the chubby and shabbily dressed security guards. I wended my way through the crowds of young, predomi-nantly African American men, and their third-tier Caucasian lawyers, still feeling like I stuck out. Some experiences never get comfortable.

There were hordes of policemen at the courthouse, mainlining doughnuts, drinking coffee, and waiting to testify. Thankfully, I didn't see Rufus. Just the thought of him was enough to make my fingers painfully throb.

Overhead, loudspeakers blared instructions, in a fuzzy, metallic voice, summoning people into the different courtrooms. "Will the parties involved in the Smith case please report to courtroom seven." I dreaded hearing the word "Grinspoon" overhead, an uncommon name, which would be recognizable to any of my patients in the courthouse, such as my patient the constable, whom I had seen during my previous visit.

I was not happy about being with Eric and not Solomon, who was tied up in a different case. When I spoke with him, Solomon seemed indifferent about the fact I had serious criminal charges hanging over my head, and the fact that I was extremely anxious about going to court without him. He assured me that I would make out just fine with Eric.

Eric's advice was "Things will turn out fine; they usually do. Try not to stress out so much." Tragically, and ironically, Eric died of a seizure in a hotel room a few months later.

This arraignment was to decide whether I was to go to trial or whether a plea deal could be worked out.

A trial was not even remotely in my interest, because I was utterly, obviously, hand-in-the-cookie-jar guilty. This would be easy to prove because I had fessed up to a lot of this stuff when initially pressured by Bruno and Rufus, and there was a paper trail of bad prescriptions I had written. A trial would almost certainly result in a criminal record, which would torpedo any future hopes of a medical career, and could possibly lead to jail time. We were not approaching the bargaining table from a position of strength.

We were hoping that after my successful stint in rehab, including a good follow-up plan and a strict monitoring program with SHP, the judge would be favorably inclined to consider me on the mend, and he would instruct the opposing counsel to cut me some slack. I still had first-offender status, because my arrest at the Nevada Test Site, during my time at Greenpeace, was dismissed by a sympathetic judge.

As we walked through the courtroom toward the bench, I thought about how at Tannenberg, I was ingrained with the idea that I had a disease, which needed to be healed. I started to lose faith that the criminal justice system would understand my transgressions as a disease, and was worried that they would view me as a selfish, malignant thug who needed correctional action. Would they throw the book at me? Treat me like a real criminal? Would it help that I was a doctor, or did that put a bull's-eye on me?

Most of all, I wanted another chance to practice primary care, with all that I had learned about myself. This didn't seem to be even on the distant horizon.

I was so anxious walking into the courtroom that my shirt started to soak through with sweat, leaving me sticky and uncomfortable, and undermining the image I was trying to project as the coolheaded, clean-cut doctor. Suddenly, this no longer seemed like a clever game that I was playing: the drugstore cowboy, hipper than thou, outsmarting the authorities, on my inflatable Greenpeace Zodiac. I didn't feel like an all-powerful doctor anymore. To say my wings had been clipped was an understatement; I just hoped the old wings wouldn't get handcuffed, chained, or permanently disabled.

The bailiffs gave me stone-faced glances, and the other defendants regarded me with cynical indifference. They had their own problems. Some of these defendants were defiant, some angry, and most looked beaten down. Many looked like zombies who had had the life sucked out of them, possibly from too many trips to the West Roxbury Municipal Courthouse. Or maybe it was too many hours spent at menial jobs. I remembered how bored and frustrated I was while working at McDonald's in high school.

The other defendants were often accompanied in court by overweight teenaged girlfriends in tight, skimpy clothing that seemed inappropriate to the venue. They clung to each other.

The female defendants were usually accompanied by tattooed, rough boy-men. This looked like tough soil for young love to sprout in.

The courtroom was stately, even ornate, though dilapidated. The mood was solemn. People were waiting for bad news. My back was aching from sitting on hard wooden seats, and I lamented the fact that I wasn't allowed to read a book, or speak, save for the occasional discreet whispers to Eric. We waited endlessly for my case to be called. I was spending $400/hour to sit on my ass, which was throbbing.

To pass the time, I tried to tune in to the other cases, a slice of life that I wouldn't ordinarily get to witness. Most of these cases seemed to be about petty theft, drug possession, or violation of custody arrangements. Several cases were related to domestic violence, and I was impressed by the courage of one young woman who stood up to her abuser. I remember thinking that she better watch her back.

I was too nervous to pay close attention, and I found myself daydreaming about taking pills again, and floating away to that blissful place, just once more, as an escape, a break from all of this suffering. I caught myself and abruptly stopped, feeling like a hypocrite. I was irrationally worried that the judge could somehow hear my thoughts, or that, just by having these thoughts, I would undermine our attempts to project my image as an earnest, reformed, contrite physician who would never, under any circumstances, do it again.

Abruptly, the courtroom became silent, and we all stood up as the judge reentered the room from his lunch break. This judge was a dour, elderly male with gray hair and a stern, no-nonsense demeanor. He didn't convey lenient, sympathetic vibes, as did my first judge.

I heard the bailiff call my name, and Eric left my side in order to have a long, animated conversation with the prosecuting attorney, just out of my earshot. I was detached, as if I were watching a movie. They conferred with the judge, who dismissed them with an abrupt nod. Suddenly, all eyes were on me. I was asked by the bailiff to stand up as they read my sentence. I held my breath, and surreptitiously crossed my fingers. "You are hereby sentenced to two years of supervised probation."

Was this good? Was I sunk? Did this mean prison? Will this ruin my career? My head was spinning, and I just stood there in stunned silence.

I didn't have time to think about it for long, or to confer with Eric, because the bailiffs immediately whisked me into a segregated area to the right of the judge, the "waiting for probation" box. I sat there as everyone in the courtroom stared at me, especially because there was a "Doctor" before my name. I felt like a bug under a magnifying glass that was about to be tortured. Please do not try to pet or feed the animals.

Vaguely I remembered from a previous conversation with Solomon that probation was a best-case outcome under the circumstances, better than CWOF. But was all probation the same? Was this what Solomon was talking about? Did our best-case scenario really involve me sitting in this box, getting gawked at by an entire courtroom of titillated spectators?

Supervised probation? Supervised by whom? My parents? Rufus? My higher power? The stone-faced bailiffs? H.? SHP? The Almighty himself? Would I still be allowed to live at home with Annie and Milo? Did I need to wear a GPS ankle bracelet to track my whereabouts? I reminded myself that I wasn't in handcuffs, or behind bars, at least not yet.

I spent an uncomfortable twenty minutes waiting and being gawked at. Then, two bailiffs escorted me downstairs to learn the terms of my probation.

Eric negotiated furiously with the probation department, and tried to get the terms of my probation to overlap with the terms of my SHP contract, so that I wouldn't have to duplicate efforts. He privately reassured me that, at the end of two years, if I strictly complied with my probation restrictions, all criminal charges would be dismissed.

The probation department required many different documents, including driver's license, proof of residence, a letter on letterhead certifying that Ben was actively seeing me as a therapist, and proof of income. They required a copy of my SHP contract and a summary from Tannenberg. After about two hours of paperwork, I said good-bye and thank you to Eric, whom I never saw again.

I was then escorted, by the burly bailiffs, to meet my probation officer. To cheer myself up, I thought, "It's a good thing they each have me by an arm, or I might make a break for it and become a fugitive from justice." I imagined these two out-of-shape, over-weight guards, who reeked of cigarette smoke, lumbering after me down the hallway, gasping for oxygen, bellowing into their radios, "We've got a doctor on the run." You can laugh, or you can cry.

I was brought back through a maze of decrepit hallways to wait in my probation officer's office. The computer on her desk looked as if it were from a prehistoric age, and the walls were plastered with bilingual advertisements for different assistance programs. SI USTED ES UNA MUJER LATINA EN RECUPERACIÓN DEL ABUSO DE SUSTANCIAS Y VIOLENCIA DOMÉSTICA, PÓNGASE EN CONTACTO CON NOSOTROS.

In walked Maria Ramirez, a heavyset, street-smart, charismatic, but jaded Latina in her midforties. She locked my gaze with distrustful eyes and spoke forcefully with a faint Hispanic accent. "If you relapse, I won't surrender you to the court, if I hear about it first from you."

"Officer Ramirez, that will *never* happen. I've learned my lesson."

"To avoid being surrendered, you need to come to monthly meetings with me, maybe more frequent. Don't be late or keep me waiting. Don't leave the state without my permission, or you might be arrested by Homeland Security. Stay out of any other kind of trouble. Don't even think of flunking a drug test."

My monthly visits to Maria involved a lot of waiting around, but I never became accustomed to being in the airless basement of the West Roxbury Municipal Courthouse. The dingy, sub-terranean waiting room was illuminated by small, dirty, barred garden windows that looked out onto piles of trash, and by fluorescent lights that blazed their way into my brain on the headache wavelength.

These visits were cognitively dissonant from the rest of my life.

My to-do list for a given day might include: Go to the market, pick up Annie or Milo from preschool, take them to a playdate, make lunches, mow the suburban lawn, and visit my probation officer. The world in which I was a successful internist, just five months previous, seemed from a different lifetime.

Waiting alongside me were gangbangers, thugs, streetwalkers, and my fellow junkies. Some had just been booked for robberies and assaults, and were there under police escort. Most had obviously been up all night, the regular office hours of thuggery. Some were high as kites and just stared vacantly or nodded off, if on heroin, or rambled on, if on meth.

Everyone looked as if this was the last place on earth they wanted to be. There was a small detention cell, with frosted windows, for violent offenders, from which occasionally rang out slurred curses and mysterious, malignant thumps against the wall.

The benches in this waiting room were close together and, as politically progressive as I consider myself to be, I was never comfortable sitting there with this subset of people. I didn't want to get mugged or knifed waiting for my probation officer. That would be too ironic. If I hadn't needed to show ID, I would have left my wallet in the car, which was slightly safer, though still quite likely to be broken into.

So that no one would talk to me or try to con me, further incriminate me, or involve me in their nefarious plans, I tried to read in peace and to surround myself with a bubble that said, "Don't bother me." I pretended to myself that I wasn't really waiting for my probation officer, but that I was a sociologist, studying all this, gathering data for a brilliant thesis.

To fit in, and avoid attention, I wanted to dress down, maybe add more bling, perhaps some loud jewelry, a nose ring, a few tattoos, a muscle shirt, but I was afraid of making a bad impression on Maria. I needed her to view me as a potentially upright citizen.

I was unable to join the conversation in the basement, because the other inhabitants spoke to each other in a "yo motherfucker, what's happening, bitch?" language that I didn't speak. There is no Rosetta stone for this language. There is no Pimsleur. There is no course at the local community college, only the school of hard knocks. In this area, I heard the N-word more than if I had been at a Ku Klux Klan rally.

I thought it best to keep my mouth shut, for fear of offending anyone or getting involved in some transaction. What really blew my cover was reading the *New England Journal of Medicine.*

Maria foiled my efforts to fastidiously avoid mixing with this criminal element by forcing me into a probation-run therapy group at the courthouse.

"Maria, are you kidding? Is this a social experiment? I've already been to rehab. I was in group therapy for about two hundred hours. I'm already in treatment with a therapist. I don't need this. Please don't make me do this."

"It will be good for you, take you down a few notches, make you less of a snob."

"It's not that I'm a snob; I just don't want to deal with these people. They are from the streets. I'm a doctor. I'm in a different category. Why should we be in treatment together? And why would you call me a snob? That's low!"

"Good-bye."

I was dismissed.

In a dank, sparsely furnished room, with bars on the windows, I sat with a bunch of other drug addicts, who looked like gang members, with lots of tattoos and jewelry, baggy jeans, and dreadlocks, and who sat in a moody gloom of tense silence. I was afraid to let out a peep.

In came a messianic, self-centered, and previously drug-addled counselor named Henry. He browbeat us to death. I started to understand why the other members of the group stared impassively into space and didn't give a shit.

Albert Einstein/Henry contended that there are no circumstances whatsoever where drug addicts should be prescribed pain medications. Even with open-heart surgery, or after a car crash, with broken bones and amputated limbs, he advocated abstinence from all sedatives and painkillers. On one's deathbed, dying an agonizing death from cancer, it's important to abstain. It was only fear of Maria that kept me sitting there and listening to him.

Henry told us he was going to go through his upcoming hip replacement without any pain medications. This was all in the great tradition of James Frey, who fabricated a dental surgery where he was supposedly tortured beyond endurance without the benefit of any pain medications. By this point, I thought that Henry deserved to be involuntarily committed to a psych unit. I lamented the fact that my medical license wasn't active, so that I could have been the one to commit him. "Oh, Henry. The ambulance is here. Time for your straitjacket."

During one group session, with no warning, Henry threw a stapler at me in order to prove that I had reflexes, to make the point that taking drugs was like a reflex to drug addicts. I was too busy ruminating over the shambles I'd made of my life to pay attention, and the stapler smashed into my knee. As I was holding my knee and hopping on one foot in a circle, howling in pain, some of the other inmates finally cracked a smile.

Jolted awake by the searing pain in my kneecap, I realized how hopelessly useless this low-end treatment was. It forced me to appreciate my rehab experience, and to admit to myself that I never would have survived if this was all that was offered to me. No wonder the others in my group seemed to have given up. Crappy lives. Crappy disease. Crappy treatment. There has to be a way to improve this.

It was not as easy as one might imagine to stay on a probation officer's good side. Staying out of trouble, in and of itself, is not enough, because they tend to be distrusting and suspicious. I thought that Maria was clinically paranoid, but, as her probation ward, I couldn't exactly refer her for a mental health consultation.

Several weeks later, as my limp from Henry's stapler was finally resolving, I was spending a peaceful evening reading at Starbucks, near my home in Hyde Park. I had secured one of the comfy armchairs and was sipping a decaf latte. I was skipping my recovery meeting, but I had to stay out until nine thirty, so that H. would believe I had been to the meeting and wouldn't torment me about having had some downtime. The nanny was home to put the kids to bed.

In walks Henry with a female friend of his, a woman of immense proportions, with a cow-like facial expression. Guiltily, I thought, "Can't addiction counselors do better than this?" The intrinsic limits of the thirteenth step. (The thirteenth step is when you pick up someone in your recovery meeting.)

As they walked in, I was deeply engrossed in *Herzog*. I didn't think much of Henry, who was at the absolute other extreme of the intellectual spectrum from Saul Bellow. I didn't feel like a rambling lecture, or AA platitudes, so I said a cursory but polite greeting and returned to my book. He nodded pleasantly, turned back to his bovine, and seemed fine with this.

The next morning, I was urgently summoned to Maria's office. I went there directly after dropping the kids off at Temple Israel preschool. Maria was livid.

"I'm disappointed in you. Henry says you were high as a kite last night at Starbucks."

"What??"

"The woman Henry was with confirmed that you were high. She said you were out of it."

"Maria, I didn't even talk to them. I was reading a book. I was reading Saul Bellow, who wouldn't make any sense if I were high. It hardly makes sense sober. I just said a brief hello to Henry. As brief and impersonal as I thought I could get away with. Frankly, I'd rather deal with anybody, rather than Henry."

"He has been a counselor here for a long time, and he is certain that you were high. I have no choice but to trust his judgment."

"Maria, go ahead and drug-test me. You are smart and savvy. You have to know that Henry is an imbecile. He's fake. And he doesn't help people. He threw a stapler at me. I'll show you the bruise."

I sat down and started pulling up the leg of my pants. Unfortunately, they were jeans and wouldn't elevate to the level of the bruise, so I started tugging in frustration.

"Stop stripping in my office. I don't care. Let's get a drug test and see who's right. It better be you and not Henry."

I passed this drug test, but her suspicion never entirely abated. In all fairness, most drug addicts, including myself, over time are more often guilty than innocent, so a suspicious attitude is probably more accurate than being universally credulous.

The next time Maria called me in abruptly was several months later, after H. called her and told her I was high. I knew there was a possibility that H. would do this, because she threatened it frequently. I believed the threats were intended to get me to comply with her household demands and stifle any rebellion.

I had called her bluff the night before, with an injudicious "Go ahead and call her. We both know you're lying. Maria won't believe you. She knows I'm not using." I was tired of being blackmailed by this threat. H. replied, "We'll see if she believes me."

H. puts on a good show. She probably sobbed into the phone and begged Maria to help her protect her children. I suppose it is possible that she truly believed I was using. Certainly she was entitled to her suspicions. In any case, the next morning, boom, I'm in Maria's office, pleading my innocence, and for my freedom.

I sat there in the basement for several hours waiting for Maria. The long wait was a deliberate component of my punishment. It just wasn't a comfortable place to wait, with the wooden benches, the fluorescent lighting, and the ambient gang members. I was irate at Maria for being so gullible, and furious at H.

Maria eventually had one of her male colleagues take me into the bathroom for a rapid drug test. He was dressed like a used-car salesman, with a frumpy sports coat and lots of hair gel. Belying his homespun demeanor, he watched me like a hawk.

This particular test has different lines on a strip, each representing a different drug. It turns bright red if you haven't used that particular drug. The test design seemed like an invitation to false positives. If the strip was expired or defective, the lines wouldn't appear, and it would look like you'd used those particular drugs.

As we were standing in the men's room watching the strip develop together, the line for marijuana was taking a long time to change color. At that point, I hadn't smoked for over a year. Maria's counterpart said, in a disarming tone of voice, like it was no big deal, "Smoked a little weed, did ya?" I heard, "About to get crucified by Maria, did ya?" I vigorously protested, and after a few more minutes of waiting, it finally came back faintly but surely negative.

It shook me up that I had come this close to being flunked by Maria. My freedom and well-being were dependent on one small red line. I wasn't comfortable with H. having that much power over my destiny.

Several weeks later, I was playing with my son, Milo, almost six years old, at our home in Hyde Park, in our sunny Victorian living room. The night before, Milo had bounded into my room. He looked up at the bottles of (legitimately prescribed) medications on my dresser, and his face darkened. In a high-pitched voice, laden with sincerity and alarm, he said, "Daddy, throw away all of those medications *right now*. We don't want you to go away again." He started sobbing.

On this afternoon, we were playing with his new toy truck on the floor. He was pretending to run over my fingers, and we were both laughing. Our game was interrupted by the doorbell. "I'll be right back, Milo."

Opening the front door, I was greeted by the suspicious visage of Maria, accompanied by two armed policemen. They were all dressed in shiny orange jackets with the word PROBATION written in large block letters on the back, just to make sure my neighbors didn't miss what was happening.

For a few moments, I was dumbfounded by this bleeding together of two incompatible parts of my life. Maria quickly explained that they were making the rounds, that this was a routine surprise visit, and that I wasn't in any trouble. She looked hugely disappointed that I wasn't caked in cocaine, smoking a spleef, or tinkering with a homegrown meth lab. There was no needle stuck into my arm, and no aroma of freshly smoked crack. Instead, it was just another boring day at the office for her.

Milo ambled over to the probation officers and flashed them a huge smile. He asked if they wanted to play with his new truck. They demurred. He thought it was the coolest thing ever that real policemen visited our house. For their part, the policemen looked embarrassed. I offered them a soda, which they politely declined.

My home situation continued to deteriorate. On several occasions, H. became so angry at me that she smashed glass jars against the wall. Above all, she couldn't stand to see me relaxing and, on several occasions, she grabbed the cup of coffee I was drinking and dumped it out, muttering that I shouldn't be "just sitting there." At other times, H. deliberately dumped my personal possessions on the floor, and kicked them around, so that I would have to gather them up.

She exploded at me because "My towel is wet." She said, "If you do the dishes, I might want to have sex." She bellowed at me, "Get me an Allegra; come to the stairs so I can tell you where it is." When she didn't like what I bought at the market, she randomly dumped the groceries into the garbage. It's fair to say that she was fraying at the edges, and that I wasn't on her good side.

She gave me endless grief for not working, even though I was collecting plenty of disability. She was working only twenty hours a week, at a women's center, for a paltry salary. She filled the rest of her time with yoga, book club, sushi lunches, and trips to the Kripalu spa in Western Massachusetts. We still had a nanny for the kids. It wasn't a bad deal for her. We had plenty of savings.

When I suggested that, much as we might pretend, this center-for-women stuff wasn't full-time "work" in a support-the-family sense, she exploded, "Get out of my house or I'll get a restraining order...I'll call SHP, and your PO, and tell them you are using... You won't get custody as an active addict."

In my diary, on October 2, 2005, after being home for less than three months: "Right now I cannot stand H.; mean, bossy, neurotic, a major bitch, controlling; I can't deal with her and I don't want to be with her I don't want to talk to her I don't want to stay married to her I'm off drugs and she's just as much of a controlling idiot. If she doesn't respect my limits it's over."

On October 8, when I hadn't yet completed the list of chores H. had given me, she locked me out in the rain for over an hour. I was so angry, I almost broke a window to get back into the cozy living room, which I could see beyond the wet pane of glass. At the last moment, I thought of Maria, her absolute edict to stay out of trouble, and how a broken window wouldn't look so good, especially with a wife who would say and do anything for revenge.

Our plan was for the four of us to drive down to New York. Annie and Milo were both proud and excited about the roles they would play in their aunt's wedding party: flower girl and ring bearer. We met at a funky Italian restaurant in Manhattan for the rehearsal dinner, which was celebratory if somewhat bland. We then drove out to Long Island in order to stay at my in-laws' house, which was empty.

My in-laws had always been supportive of me and my attempts at recovery. They sent me an orange sweater (orange again!) when I was at rehab, which touched me to the core, even if I would never wear a sweater that practically broiled my skin and made me look like the Great Pumpkin. Their gift symbolized that both sides of the family cared about what happened to me, regardless of the fights between H. and myself.

My in-laws assured us that their house was "safe," with no controlled substances lying around. We arrived there at about eleven p.m., after the rehearsal dinner. We put Annie and Milo to sleep, followed shortly by H., who was out cold, snoring and muttering, after a full day of driving and dealing with family politics. I was utterly wired.

Being awake and alone in the early hours of the morning is a common space where addicts get into trouble. I had discussed my recovery in detail with my in-laws. They knew I was still in early recovery and needed, at all costs, to avoid temptation.

Unfortunately, old habits die hard. I tiptoed up into the attic, where I used to surreptitiously smoke pot, but the pipe and small bag I had stashed there had been cleaned out. Next, following some primitive addict instinct, I started rooting around in the back of the medicine cabinet closest to the master bedroom. Nothing good has *ever* come from my snooping around in medicine cabinets. (I've since heard of people putting marbles in their medicine closets during parties, to prevent theft of drugs. The marbles would make a huge noise as they rolled out of the medicine cabinet and started bouncing around.)

Deeply buried, under all sorts of ointments, liniments, shampoos, soaps, shaving creams, and bottles of Tylenol and Advil, was a full prescription bottle of Vicodin.

Everything I had learned during ninety days of rehab was displaced by an unexpected rush of euphoria. All thoughts, sense, and accumulated wisdom were circumvented by my body's anticipation of what was to come next. My heart was happily palpitating.

The next memory I have is being in the front seat of the car, driving into Manhattan for the wedding, with H. screaming at me for being intoxicated. I was denying it, though I remember struggling my absolute hardest just to keep my eyes open, thinking, "If I can keep my eyes open, this will be fine."

I gradually sobered up enough to participate in the wedding, a yuppie festival, which was held at an opulent riverside function room. The kids and I watched all kinds of luxury boats steaming or sailing up and down the Hudson River. H. said, "At least you do sober up quickly." I danced clumsily with the bride, was competently in charge of the kids, and was even able to get them back to the hotel we had moved to without mishap.

During the wedding, I had enough sense not to give the toast I had planned, which sounded witty, teasing, and sentimental when I composed it, but which would have come out awkward and insulting in front of hundreds of people, with the delivery slurred by drugs.

But the damage was done. In my diary from that night: "Fuck—I used and H. knows I used. God damn it, a blackout... God damn it, after all this crap, I'm under stress and I use (I CAN'T have a positive test. No sanction for dilute tests). Blackout from Sea Cliff to NYC—only one recollection, of H. driving, yelling at me, me trying my hardest to keep my eyes open."

My first call was to Lyle, my best friend from rehab, whom I was still in frequent touch with.

"Hi, Lyle, how's things? Are you in prison yet?"

"No, Grinspoon, things are real good. I'm back to work, and me and the wife are doing better. What's new in Boston? Everything OK? You still clean and sober?"

"Um, not really. I had a major slipup. I took some Vicodin last night, and all hell's about to break loose."

"That was stupid! What happened?"

"It was unexpected. All of a sudden it was in front of me. I didn't think, I just swallowed a bunch of pills. Next thing I know, I'm in a car, with H. screaming at me, trying to wake up for her sister's wedding."

"Oh, shit. That must have done wonders for spousal relations."

"I'm screwed with the board too. They were just about to consider my case. And my probation officer is going to shoot me."

"Grinspoon, I know you don't want to hear this, but I think you better call Nate right away and get his advice. Otherwise they are going to fry your ass."

"OK, Lyle, and thanks. Nice knowing you."

In a panic, I called Nate at Tannenberg. He said, "Grinspoon, I'm sorry to hear this, but I'm really proud of you for telling me. The important thing, right now, is to lessen the chance of a repeat, and not to worry about the other stuff."

"It's easy for you to say this; you won't have Maria dismembering you in the dungeon of the courthouse."

"I hate to say this, Grinspoon, but been there and done that. It will be OK. Go to a meeting tonight."

He reminded me that back when he was in my shoes, he had been in jail, and this shut me up. I still wasn't looking forward to dealing with Maria, or even Solomon.

Nate suggested I approach all of the involved third parties—SHP, Ben, my psychiatrist, my attorney, and Maria—with honesty, as the best way to mitigate what I had done, and to refocus myself on my recovery. He said they all know that these things happen quite frequently in early recovery, and would be somewhat understanding.

Nate then suggested I come back to Tannenberg for three to four days, but I resisted this; it felt too much like an admission of utter failure. What else could they teach me that I hadn't learned in ninety days?

I saw a different side of Maria that day, almost a compassionate side. She said, "Try not to beat yourself up too much. This happens all the time. Because you told me yourself, I'm not going to surrender you to the judge. But you are going to have to come see me more frequently." SHP made me re-sign my contract, and increased my testing frequency.

In terms of the medical board, the timing of this slip couldn't have been worse. In his office, Solomon and I hunkered down into damage-control mode. Solomon started off on the topic of H.: "What is your wife doing? She's undermining us. She's gone off the reservation." H.'s actions, by calling SHP, the medical board, and Maria, were running directly counter to our efforts. Solomon said, "Regardless of your situation, or hers, it's in her interest for you to go back to work. If you are married, if you are divorced, she needs you to work."

"Solomon, she's angry and hurt. We're having problems. There's nothing I can do about this."

Solomon informed me that he was communicating with the investigators from the medical board. He said that I needed to call our former nanny Ruth, in New Zealand, to tell her what had happened, and to tell her to expect a call from him.

I knew that Ruth and her dad had been questioned by the police in New Zealand as a result of my writing and picking up prescriptions in her name. I told Solomon that I was too embarrassed and felt too guilty to call her. I asked him to try to leave her out of this as much as possible, even if it damaged our case. She was a fundamentally innocent and unknowing victim, and I didn't want to make things worse for her.

When I asked Solomon to summarize where things stood, he sympathetically grimaced and said, "We have a rocky road ahead of us with the medical board; there was a criminal charge, though pretrial probation is better than CWOF, you had a relapse, and most importantly, there was patient involvement. I would have pushed for one year with SHP or six months documented sobriety, but now [with the relapse at Brittney's wedding] the board needs more than six months starting now. The best case is one year from the day the new SHP contract was signed."

Solomon said that a more likely scenario was that the board would insist upon a minimum of eighteen months of documented sobriety, starting from the August 2005 relapse. I wouldn't be able to start looking for work until February 2007, almost two years from when I last took care of a patient. This dismal scenario assumed that someone would hire me after all that time on the sidelines and with such a dark stain on my record. It was hard not to agree with Solomon's previous assessment, "You are a major-league screwup."

Solomon's challenge was to present my situation to the board in the best possible light. As he had just bleakly surmised, things weren't going so well along these lines. They might throw away the key for good if I flunked any more drug tests. We weren't entirely sure there still was a key, given the "patient involvement" in my addiction. In addition to flawless compliance with my SHP contract, we needed a game-changer, something to convince them that I had gained insight into the error of my ways. Solomon had just the ticket.

*   *   *

Solomon enrolled me in a two-day-long program called Professional/
Problem-Based Ethics (ProBE) in New Jersey. According to their
website:

> The ProBE Program is the original educational interven-
> tion in ethics for all healthcare professionals under disci-
> pline by their licensing boards or other oversight agencies.
> We provide education for ethics violations or unprofessional
> conduct secondary to boundary violations in the practice of
> health care…including, but not limited to, sexual miscon-
> duct, drug diversion, and inappropriate use of social media;
> misrepresentation or falsification of credentials; financial
> irregularities; disruptive behavior; civil or criminal viola-
> tions; or failure to adequately inform patients in obtaining
> consent.

It made me feel better that there were all of these other devi-
ant things that doctors had done that I hadn't even thought of
doing. At least I wasn't the only one in trouble.

While driving down to New Jersey, I listened to "Lose Yourself" by Eminem, which channeled the anger I felt at having to
attend this demeaning seminar on how to be an appropriate doctor. It felt like preschool: "Now, Peter, that's not an appropriate
way to behave. Use your big-boy voice."

The ProBE seminar took place on the campus of one of the
large universities in New Jersey. The rooms had fireplaces,
exposed brick, and bookshelves stuffed and overflowing with
classic literature. I always salivate at the sight of books. Even
more than with opiates. Under other circumstances, being here
would have pleasantly reminded me of my Swarthmore days,
when we sat around and philosophized until one in the morning
and, after, compared notes on what we were planning on reading
next. I imagined myself sliding into one of the comfy chairs with
a whole stack of novels, and reading the weekend away.

The two course leaders were skinny and effete, had spectacles, and spoke with showy, nasal Ivy League intonations. They used complex jargon to impress us with how learned they were. "The difference between constitutional morality and intrinsic morality…" I studied moral philosophy in college, so I knew these words, and I knew that there were much less pretentious ways to express the same ideas. Still, I was a captive audience.

I didn't think either of these professors would survive very long on their own, in the state of nature, or, for that matter, anywhere outside of an academic environment. They would be clubbed senseless by the first caveman they ran into. They seemed overly specialized.

At the seminar, there were nine other participants, but I was the only drug addict. Some were there for financial violations— Medicare fraud or tax evasion. A few were there for medical records and privacy (HIPAA) violations. One physician assistant had opened the chart of her ex-boyfriend's new girlfriend, searching for angry ammunition.

Several participants had crossed sexual lines with their patients. One surgeon's wife attended this conference with her husband to ensure that, this time around, he understood why it's wrong to continue to sleep with patients. She talked about his "disease" and his "addiction" but, to me, he was clearly just a macho sleazeball.

I didn't think that any of the other attendees, except for the jilted physician assistant, were genuinely contrite about what they had done. They mostly looked unhappy that they had been busted and that they couldn't continue to get away with what they were getting away with. No more padding bank accounts or screwing patients. Like me, they were primarily there at the suggestion of their attorneys.

The content of the seminar included lots of talk about "duties," "intrinsic values," and "constitutive rules," all of which I had managed to violate while feeding my addiction.

I came into ProBE thinking that I had nothing to learn and would go through the motions in order to help Solomon make me look good. By the end, I wasn't so sure that it was a waste of time. The scenarios presented were thought-provoking and complex. It wasn't always clear what the right thing to do was.

Driving home, I felt that I had a much broader perspective about where my interactions with patients had gone off track. While it was taking place, with boundaries being eroded little by little, a pill traded here and stolen there, with willing coconspirators, I hadn't noticed. When viewed retrospectively, in the context of the entire spectrum of violated boundaries and harm inflicted, I was able to clearly glimpse a much uglier version of my past actions.

Deep down, I had always believed that, at some point, the criminal charges filed against me would be dismissed. Dr. T., Dr. Stern, Nate, and countless others I had encountered on my path had been in similar trouble and had clawed their way out. My crimes were clearly done in the context of an addiction, which I was treating. Only a few people I encountered had actually been to prison, and those were for extreme violations, like selling prescriptions to undercover cops, or federal trafficking of methamphetamine.

Whether I would ever wield a stethoscope again, and be allowed to heal people, was entirely another matter. The mere thought of dealing with the medical board gave me palpitations.

Having just spent three days at ProBE vividly analyzing my boundary violations with a newfound clarity, I was dubious the medical board would even consider letting me back into medicine. "Dr. Grinspoon, we've considered your case carefully, and would suggest that you find something else to do with your life." I wasn't even sure that I would ever let myself back to work, if I were on the board.

The board was still freezing me out, so I had plenty of time to hurry up and wait.

On April 19, 2006, after a sequence of spectacular arguments and lots of smashed ceramic objects, H. kicked me out of the house, as it turned out, for the final time. She said to Annie, who had just turned six, "Daddy is leaving. He's not doing well with the medicines." When I protested to H. that it was my house too, so she didn't have the authority to kick me out into the street, she replied, "I'll say I'm worried about my safety."

I pointed out that, save for the one relapse at the wedding, my recovery was going quite well. I had apologized profusely to anyone that would listen, and even to those who wouldn't. I argued to H. that she should understand, from Al-Anon, that recovery wasn't always a linear process. My arguments fell on deaf ears. We never lived under the same roof again.

Over the next several months, as it became clear that we were getting divorced, we had to unite in order to find a way to communicate this to Annie and Milo. The four of us sat in the living room of our Hyde Park house for a "family meeting." Annie and Milo were sitting on either side of me, snuggled up on the sofa. H. was sitting in the comfy recliner just adjacent to the sofa, but she was sitting up ramrod straight, and her body language was that of a very tense person. She was loudly drumming her fingers.

Annie and Milo then heard the words that all kids must instinctively dread, "Mom and I have decided to get a divorce." In unison, all four of us started sobbing.

We explained that I would be moving out permanently and living with my parents. We tried to put a positive face on things, and reminded them that I'd still be very nearby. Kids are intuitive, and they knew that this spelled some not yet fully understood doomsday scenario.

In the face of their tears, H. managed "You'll see Dad a lot." (Oh, what a hypocrite! How she tried to limit my time with them. I suspected she tried to restrict my access so as to increase child support.)

The home atmosphere had become so polluted with animosity, yelling, accusations, and door slamming, that our concerted attempts at reassurance didn't sound credible even to two credulous young children, who weren't yet old enough to be skeptical of adults.

According to my diary on April 30, 2006, "Not living at home, H. preventing me from seeing them. A and M call (breaks my heart) are you sick? Are you getting better? Are you doing what you need to do? Annie asked, 'Can we visit you? Mom says it's OK if you show her what she needs to see' (i.e. negative drug test). [H.] gets kids hopes up as a way to control my behavior."

The original conditions on my seeing the kids were that I show H. a negative drug screen and that I don't drive them. Other conditions soon started to appear. By early May, "You can only see the children after you agree to clean up the house."

I believe that, at the time, H. had expected to punish me by kicking me out for a few weeks, as she had done before, and then letting me back in, chastened, diminished, and obedient. I don't think it even occurred to her that I might have the gumption to leave the marriage, even if I hadn't always been a doormat.

I believe that H. loved me in the same way that Salamano, a character in *The Stranger* by Albert Camus, loved his dog. Salamano routinely beat and abused this dog, but when the dog died, he was utterly lost and bereft.

From my perspective, I knew that it had been a long time since I'd felt nurtured in our marriage. Intermittently, there was affection, and fun, and socializing, and vacations, and adventures, and we had plenty of money. In the spaces in between, I was mostly getting criticized for not doing chores correctly, or being punished for not submitting to her often contradictory whims. A general sense of peacefulness and contentment had been eluding me, possibly ever since we tied the knot.

I had always been afraid to be on my own, partially due to being "abandoned" by my brother Danny dying when I was seven. This neurotic fear has led me into many ridiculous and unfulfilling relationships, dating at least back to Tami in medical school, whose family helped start me on the Vicodin. This fear of aloneness is part of what kept me in the marriage.

I knew that children of divorce didn't usually do as well as their peers, and I was concerned about what would happen to Annie and Milo if our family split apart. I had anxieties about divorce and the unknown, child support, custody, alimony, lawyers, courtrooms, litigation, and long separations from the children. These fears, too, kept me in the marriage.

With pills, I could convince myself that I was happy enough to leave my family intact. I was too passive and discombobulated to change my life circumstances even if I wanted to. I could put up with *some* crap for the sake of Annie and Milo. Couldn't I? Don't all parents sacrifice for their kids?

Without the drugs, it was a different ball game. Separated from the kids, sleeping in my old bedroom in my parents' house, the bedroom that used to be Danny's, I stayed up at night staring at the posters that my brother Danny had plastered to the wall. One was of a Hassidic rabbi in a telephone booth, changing into a Superman outfit. Danny had put a sticker with the label KOSHER over his crotch.

Looking at Danny's effects, many unused for three decades, kept like museum pieces by my parents, it was hard not to feel that life is short and uncertain. Who says that I need to continue to shackle myself to someone who rarely was even nice to me? Fifty percent of marriages end in divorce, and the divorced people I knew seemed to be doing OK; some, in fact, seemed quite happy with their new leases on life.

I questioned whether anything, divorce included, could be as bad for Annie and Milo as what they were currently witnessing, our constant fighting, anger, and accusations.

I realized that our marriage was incompatible with my continued recovery. We had been stuck in a destructive feedback cycle, which brought out the worst qualities in both of us. I would tune out, she would get angry, I'd tune out some more, with or without drugs, and she'd get even angrier. She hadn't given me any credit or positive reinforcement.

Above all, I was angry. I felt that she had been dumping on me because I couldn't fund her lifestyle of nannies, book clubs, pedicures, and the gym scene. What about sticking together through thick and thin? I was tired of being kicked around. Riding a sustained burst of indignation, I obtained the name of an attorney from my twin brother Martin, and filed for divorce.

For my seminal meeting with the medical board, Solomon advised me to "dress and act like a doctor." Am I supposed to wear a stethoscope? My white lab coat? Should I walk up to the board members and take their pulse? Hit their kneecaps with my reflex hammer? Tell them to exercise more and lose some of their extra fat?

The idea of being confronted with what I had done, by an attorney for the medical board, was enough to burn an ulcer through the full thickness of my esophagus. There are no antacids in existence that are strong enough for dealing with the medical board.

Once again, we descended to the basement offices, and they brought us into a small, stifling room with no windows, glaring fluorescent lights, and a stark metal table in the center. I sat next to Solomon, wanting to hide behind him, or crawl under the table, away from the lights. Hiding under the table wouldn't qualify as acting like a doctor.

An investigator and an attorney for the board were sitting directly opposite us. In my mind, they were salivating and sharpening their fangs.

The investigator was a middle-aged, slightly overweight woman with brown hair and warm eyes. She had a kindly smile, and she nodded encouragingly when I responded to their questions. In sharp contrast, the board's attorney was humorless, abrupt, unfriendly, and businesslike—a shark. He acted as if he was on television and had a wide audience. He grilled me for two and a half hours.

In principle, I wanted to be entirely open and honest with the board, and to put this all behind me once and for all. But I was also apprehensive about the type of grave I would be digging for myself. What mattered most to me at the time was getting back to work, so that I could start to do good again.

I was mired in a prisoner's dilemma. On the one hand, any information I volunteered would contribute to the brutal case they were building against me. On the other hand, anything I didn't tell them, but which they found out about independently, would be far more damaging, and would delay my return to work even more, if not permanently.

As Solomon had explained earlier, "The board is aware that what they know about you is only the tip of the iceberg. This is true for most criminals, unless they happen to be caught during their first crime."

The board's agenda was to make as detailed a case against me as possible, to support whatever action they ultimately decided to take. This meant drilling as deep as they could.

Their attorney kept pressing me, "You have to tell us which patients you shared drugs with. You have to tell us their names. Otherwise, we can't confirm anything you are saying."

This was problematic. There weren't any complaints against me. There weren't any lawsuits. I wanted to keep it that way. I didn't want the board contacting these patients, stirring up trouble, reopening old wounds, and vastly compounding my problems.

Solomon sharply rebutted, "Why would my client make any of this stuff up? So that he can get himself in more trouble? You only know about any of this because my client has been so forthcoming in the first place. The names don't matter, and we're not going to give them to you. We want to leave these people out of it. What matters is that Dr. Grinspoon is getting treatment and is doing well." With this, they let it go.

The conversation segued to how my addiction began. Without using names, I briefly narrated what had transpired with Tami and her father, and the enormous supply of Vicodin he gave us. The investigator turned bright red and looked like she was going to have a stroke. She said, "He's still practicing in Massachusetts? Don't tell me this; I don't want to hear it. This kind of thing keeps me up at night."

The board's attorney wanted me to implicate friends and colleagues who, if anything, were unwitting victims of my drug-seeking manipulations. They wanted to know about anyone I hit up for a prescription under the guise of a "migraine." There was no way I was going to get anyone else in trouble, beyond what I had originally mentioned to Bruno and Rufus when they ambushed and pressured me in my office. I had already caused too much mayhem in people's lives. This was entirely my fault, not theirs, and there was no reason to drag them into the morass.

After two and a half hours of this, Solomon, my splitting migraine, and I climbed back out of the basement. Even the polluted air of Roxbury was refreshing after being in that basement. We climbed into Solomon's Lexus convertible to zip back to his office. By then, I had probably contributed leather seats and new brake pads.

I was discouraged about my prospects of returning to work as a doctor and, in my diary, tried to convince myself that I didn't even want to go back. "Fuck the board with them being so strict re: letting me do something no one else wants to do [primary care] with less money and more stress. I can let someone else do the rectal exams." The doctor doth protest too much. I was desperate to return to work.

At that night's physician recovery meeting, I urgently needed to regain perspective and hope. I was part of a group of thirty recovering physicians who were sitting around a table, eating a dinner of limp cold cuts and bitter coffee in one of the conference rooms of the Medical Society of Massachusetts. We use only first names, to protect privacy.

One participant was a self-proclaimed sex addict who retained escorts when traveling to medical conferences. That is, until his wife found out by reading his credit card receipts. I wondered if he was using the guise of "addict" to get out of trouble with his wife. "Honey, I have been fucking the nanny for the last two years, but it's only because of my sex addiction, a disease that requires understanding and compassion, and now I'm in recovery."

I thought of all the swindlers who attended the ProBE professional ethics conference in New Jersey. They could have claimed that they were addicted to money, and used the "it's a disease that I'm not in control of" defense. People shouldn't be allowed to exploit the concept of "being an addict" to explain any and all types of bad behavior.

As with all recovery meetings, the participants ranged from shaky, self-conscious newcomers, sober for mere days, just about to leave for rehab, to wise and well-grounded old-timers. I could see myself, a year earlier, in the cloudy, defiant, uncertain expressions of the newbies.

It is unique that all of the participants at this meeting were physicians or dentists. Yes, docs have the same problems that everyone else has. Diabetes, alcoholism, depression. Meth addiction. Divorce. Suicide. Nonetheless, everyone expects from us a robotic consistency at all times. When a doctor screws up, it's a big scandal, and the news coverage is utterly devoid of compassion. The subtext is "fuckup, selfish, loser doctor." To know the people in this room is to know compassion, but this gets lost in the shuffle.

To get the conversation started, a nasally sounding anesthesiologist began reading from the Narcotics Anonymous book: "Addiction is a disease that involves more than the use of drugs. Some of us believe that our disease was present long before the first time we used."

If I weren't smack-dab in the middle of it, it would have been a bizarre concept: dozens of well-dressed and bespectacled physicians reading from the Narcotics Anonymous handbook. In prior circumstances, I would have associated this book with homeless street druggies who broke into houses, stole cars, injected heroin and coke, shared needles, and slept under bridges, not with the clean-cut and responsible doctors we all see in the course of our daily lives.

Not everyone gets to witness the director of a high-powered internal-medicine practice sincerely discuss humility, or a wealthy and venerated neurosurgeon extol the virtues of powerlessness and letting go (and letting God). If the god of stereotypes sat in on this meeting, he would lose his abilities. These meetings helped me start to believe again that people can grow and change for the better.

What stuck out the most during the meetings was the exquisite guilt and shame that these doctors felt, and the sincerity of their remorse and their motivation to make amends to their patients. None of them intended to do harm to anyone, especially not to their patients. The ones who had returned to practice were flourishing.

I raised my hand. "This morning I was at the medical board

with my attorney. They were gunning for me. With good reason, but it was excruciating. I now have a new ulcer, so excuse
me if I start to hemorrhage. They asked me about sharing medications with patients. I didn't know how much to tell them,
and they kept tripping me up. They didn't seem like advocates
of the disease model. This was straight-up crime and punishment. They are never going to let me back to work, and this is
just so discouraging."

"Peter, I went through the same thing eight years ago. Don't
take this personally; they are a bureaucracy, who are overly concerned with covering themselves. We are priorities when we crash
and burn, but it's true that getting impaired physicians back to
work, even if they are sober, is a low priority for them." Another
colleague said, "It always seems hopeless right after meeting with
the board, but things die down. If you stay sober, keep putting
one foot in front of the other, this will die down." They echoed
Dr. Stern's message: "If you just don't do drugs, everything will
work itself out." I had no choice but to trust them.

True to these predictions, it took the board months to get back to
Solomon. On August 15, 2006, seventeen months after my last
day of work, I spoke with Solomon over the phone. "The board is
in no hurry. You can approach them for a very restricted license
if you have an entirely nonclinical job lined up. The shortest
possible time frame would be eighteen months from your 8/05
relapse, which would be 2/07, but realistically they might want
to wait for three years."

Three years??? Gulp. At that point, would I even remember
how to take a blood pressure? If I waited that long, would they
say that too much time had passed, and that I needed to retrain?
Retraining programs are expensive, time-consuming, and humiliating. Would I have to repeat residency?

What's an entirely "nonclinical" job? Please not Home Depot!
That would make H. too happy. Back to my high school job at
McDonald's? "Hi, I'm Dr. Grinspoon, would you like some
fries with that burger?" This didn't sound good. Neither my

cholesterol nor my self-esteem would ever recover from another stint at McDonald's.

Solomon explained that the board was concerned with covering itself against charges of leniency, and that they err on the side of caution when protecting the public. He reminded me that their position was not entirely ungrounded, given my checkered history.

Solomon acknowledged that it's a catch-22 to look for a job without a medical license in order to show the board that I had a job lined up and in order to petition to get my license back. To a prospective employer, I'd have to say, "I might have my medical license back if you offer me a job." Solomon said, "The board knows this but they don't give a shit."

In October 2006, Solomon told me that there was a meeting with the board on November 1, and that I would definitely get a suspension because of my prescription violations and because of sharing prescriptions with patients.

The news of my upcoming suspension hit me hard. I truly felt like I didn't have anything to look forward to. I was dealing with too much at once, trying to recover and trying to be a newly separated dad under near-impossible circumstances. It's heart-wrenching to watch your own kids suffer. Annie was becoming quieter and was prone to anxiety at group events such as birthday parties. One day, when I picked her up from school, she said, "I hate Annie."

I was also dealing with the courts, probation, SHP, the medical board, taking drug tests, driving to meetings, all while dealing with an increasingly vicious divorce. There's only so much a given person can take at once.

Living with my parents was depressing, even though they couldn't possibly have been more kind and supportive. Not working was depressing. Visiting Maria in the basement of the courthouse was depressing. Peeing into a cup every week was depressing. I was lonely, having lost all social contact at work and much of my social network to the divorce. H. encouraged people to take sides. They were with her or against her. Under pressure, friends and acquaintances stepped away from both of us.

Some friends and my close-knit group of cousins were still around, but I suffered from a newfound embarrassment and awkwardness around them, due to feeling ashamed of having taken medications from them, or of wrecking my life and letting them down.

I was so lonely, I decided to start dating. To quote Green Day, "When masturbation's lost its fun / You're fucking lonely." I knew that loneliness was a major trigger for my addiction, and I needed companionship, though hopefully not to rush headlong into another disastrous relationship.

Without work or new friends, the Internet is hands down the best way to meet people. A critical part of Internet dating is developing a narrative that shines a favorable light on one's personality and activities, so that attractive people will take the bait and want to meet up with you. Participants list their attractive attributes, and if the important boxes are checked off, two people decide to meet in person.

I had a difficult time packaging, in an attractive manner, the sum total of my addiction, my divorce, my lack of employment and money, the criminal charges, and the fact that I was living with my parents. I really didn't have much to work with. The MD helped, but even then I had to explain that it was actually suspended for the time being, and I wasn't practicing.

My bio would read something like this:

Drug addict doctor, with suspended medical license, enmeshed in vicious divorce, with two small children, living with my parents, with criminal charges hanging over my head, and broke, looking for anything remotely female that is desperate enough to spend a minute or two with me before running in the opposite direction.

To complicate matters around this time, mid-2007, after suspending me, the medical board sent out a detailed press release describing the infractions they had uncovered in their investigation. Most discerning Internet daters are savvy enough to Google the stranger they are about to meet. When the name Peter Grinspoon was Googled, this press release was the first thing that came up.

On several occasions, dates were abruptly canceled. One woman, a successful author, called a few hours before we were to meet and said, "I wish you the best but I just can't go forward with this." We were just going to meet for coffee. It's not as if I was proposing marriage. Another, a psychiatrist, who had enthusiastically e-mailed me for weeks, disappeared and blocked her e-mail.

Shirley was a woman who I wish had taken the time to Google me, but didn't. I was reading *The Road* by Cormac McCarthy, which was so bleak, it made my life circumstances seem better in comparison. I had arrived early, was seated, and was trying to guess which woman Shirley was, among the steady string of attractive, unaccompanied women walking through the door to Starbucks.

Eventually, a tall, brown-haired woman with leathery skin came in and started looking for someone who resembled my online picture. As our conversation progressed, I asked her what kind of law she practiced. Knowing I was a physician, Shirley joked, "I didn't want to scare you off, so I didn't tell you earlier, but I work for the medical board." *This can't be happening.*

Stunned, I was at a rare and complete loss for words. Wondering if she had read my file, or was working on my case, I eventually replied, "That's great. What exactly do you do for the medical board?"

"I prosecute doctors who break the law, don't practice up to standard, or who are on drugs."

At this point, any hypothetical hope of romance had vanished, due to mutual conflict of interest, but we had an interesting and meaningful conversation.

"It's actually been quite stressful dealing with the board. The other attorney seems overly aggressive. I feel that they are trying to nail me, and aren't really participating with SHP in order to help me overcome my addiction and get back to work. It all seems for show."

"*I'm actually looking for other jobs, because the medical board is too disorganized and ineffectual.*"

We hugged good-bye.

Not knowing when I'd be allowed to return to work, not equipped for any other type of work, I was determined to make the best use I could of this time, by reading as much literature as I could, working out, and focusing on my kids. Somewhere down there was still the enthusiastic Peter who could turn any lemons into lemonade, and who would come out of this entire mud pile on top.

In rehab, Nate had encouraged us to discover the parts of ourselves that existed separately from our identities as physicians. At the time, that sounded great. Doctors are people too, with hobbies, interests, and whole facets of our personality that get buried under the work and the pressure.

In reality, try as I may, my life felt empty when I wasn't practicing primary care. Sometimes you don't know that you miss something until it's gone. Like Salamano and his dog.

Primary care had been my sole focus for twelve years, starting in medical school. It was an entire state of being, and was an impossible void to fill. It was my mission in life, coming after Greenpeace. Try as I might to convince myself that I didn't really want to deal with smelly, grumpy, needy, manipulative people all day, I missed it horribly.

I fought to maintain a positive attitude, but the details of my current predicament, battling with H., feeling shame, waking up in my parents' house, hardly seeing the kids, settled like a dark cloud and tainted everything I did, from spending time with Annie and Milo to going to the gym or reading all of the books I had stacked up in precarious piles by my bed.

The main symbol of this dark cloud was the need to go to my old office at the Faulkner Hospital in order to pick up my belongings, such as my medical textbooks, my favorite Starbucks coffee mug, and my photographs of Annie and Milo. I suspected that my stethoscope had gathered a thick layer of dust, if not rust, from having been idle for so long. I put this task off as long as possible, because I was unable to face my former colleagues.

I knew that these colleagues, after they got over the inconvenience of caring for my three thousand patients, on short notice, were rooting for me to regain my health, but I couldn't bring myself to face them. I couldn't bring myself to say what I felt, something like, "Sorry you had to take all of my calls and do all of my paperwork because I fucked up my life."

Because of the press release from the medical board, everyone in the office—medical assistants, secretaries, nurses—knew what had happened. They would piece together the lies and my bizarre behavior, my late-night returns to the office, the missing medication samples. These were the people who had searched my desk and locked me out of the office. I was in disgrace, and it was difficult to face.

Every so often, I would receive a message on my answering machine: "Hi, this is Susan from Primary Care Internal Medicine Associates. We hope you are doing well. Also, we would like to schedule a time for you to come by and pick up your possessions." Mature, responsible adult that I was, I ignored and erased the messages.

It wasn't until two years had passed that I went, with my twin brother Martin, to gather my office possessions, which had been boxed up and moved to a dank security shed in the basement of the adjacent parking garage. My dermatology book was missing, and several of the photographs of Annie and Milo were wrinkled or bent in their box, a far cry from the proud spot they used to have on the door of my office. There was dust on my diplomas, and my stethoscope looked flaccid.

We solemnly loaded these remnants of my medical career into my Subaru, drove them away, and stored them in a dark corner of the basement of my parents' home, where they could continue to molder until the end of time.

*   *   *

Ever since my relapse at Brittney's wedding, SHP was all over me, with frequent urine tests and strict warnings against drinking too much water before these tests. Dr. Stern told me to limit my liquid consumption to no more than eight ounces on the morning of a test. That wasn't even a full cup of coffee.

Tightening the screws further, they announced a new requirement for a hair test, which, in theory, tested for any drug use during the last three to six months. This had to be completed within one week's time.

This new requirement sent me into an absolute panic, even though there wasn't any drug use to speak of besides my relapse at Brittney's wedding, which they already knew all about. A positive hair test would absolutely torpedo me with the medical board, with the courts, and with my custody situation, even if it took place in the context of drug use I had already admitted to. I wasn't taking any chances.

I read what I could find on the efficacy and false-positive rates of the hair tests, and I got the sense that they weren't as effective as they were touted to be. A drug needed to be used three times in order to build up sufficient residue in the hair follicle to be detectable. That meant mine would be clean.

I still wasn't taking any chances. On the Internet, I came across a plethora of "cures" for a looming hair test, including elixirs and shampoos that were advertised as able to clean the hair of all drug residue.

On a practical level, I had no way of knowing if any of these hair-cleansing products actually worked. I had too much at stake to trust the claims of fly-by-night drug-culture Internet sites, yet I didn't expect to come across a *Consumer Reports* issue addressing this particular product.

SHP warned me not to cut my hair too short and not to bleach it before the test, because that destroyed their ability to detect. In some states, bleaching hair right before a hair test is considered contempt of court, a criminal offense.

I wasn't restricted from washing my hair, and from what I had learned, each time I shampooed I would dislodge a few molecules here and there, out of the limited number of molecules they were trying to detect in the first place. I spent the next several days scrubbing my hair in the mildew-encrusted showers at Gold's Gym, because at home, the hot water would run out after about ten minutes. At Gold's, it was unlimited.

The place I had to go to for my hair test was a good hour away, in Lynn, Massachusetts, at Willow Laboratories, run by a toxicology specialist, Dr. Picante. Driving up there, I nervously picked at my scalp, which was itchy and irritated from the four days of shampooing it had just endured. My hair was so dry, it felt disconnected and alien, like some radioactive rug with a mind of its own, intent on getting me into trouble.

I could picture the remaining molecules of Vicodin barricaded in the hair follicles, dug in, holding out, willing themselves to wreck my life, jeering at me, "We're still here, you motherfucker. We're not giving up. Remember the Alamo!"

Willow Laboratories is located in a dingy neighborhood adjacent to the Lynn Community Health Center, but as I entered the foyer, everything seemed modern and clean. After filling out my initial paperwork, I waited for about an hour in a lobby filled with shady-looking teenagers who were addicted to oxy or meth. Their pissed-off, druggie-cool attitude reminded me of Maria's basement.

Eventually, I was ushered into a lab room by an ungainly Asian American lab tech sporting a poorly fitting lab coat. Intently focused on the business at hand, refractory to my attempts at humor and small talk, he unceremoniously snipped several different small locks of my hair and sealed them in a sterile container. My fate seemed to be sealed in that sterile plastic container as well.

After the hair test, I looked like a mental patient, with asymmetric chunks of hair snipped out, down to my scalp. I was unable to reach my recovery-buddy barber, to see if he could spruce things up. At home, my mom, not one to criticize, said, "Peter, they gave you a *terrible* haircut."

After weeks of nervous waiting, I received the result of my hair test: negative. Speaking with SHP over the phone, I was like, "I told you so. Why would you paranoid bureaucrats have suspected an innocent person like me in the first place?" Inwardly, I was profoundly relieved. This felt like a new lease on life, another chance. I knew that the chances wouldn't keep coming indefinitely.

My new girlfriend, Sarah, was a pediatric nurse with low self-esteem. She spent five hours a week in old-fashioned psychoanalysis, where she lay on a couch and free-associated to a snoozing analyst, in order to overcome the trauma of being left by her husband. I urged her to switch to a more modern flavor of psychotherapy, as psychoanalysis is generally useless and outdated, but I think she mostly craved the social interaction with the analyst, pricey as it was.

Sarah's mom suffered from arthritis and, while visiting, left a big bottle of the opiate painkiller Darvon in the bathroom in her medicine bag, unzipped, sitting on the back of the toilet. I removed these preternaturally large pink pills from the prescription bottle, held them in my hand, and counted them.

Drug addicts hold their nose when dealing with Darvon, because it is weak and doesn't have much effect. Using it is like forcing a European who is used to rich ale to drink Bud Light. A gambler addicted to hundred-dollar slots can get only so excited about five-cent slots. (Darvon has since been removed from the market because it can cause lethal heart arrhythmias.)

I knew I wouldn't have a drug test coming up for at least four days, because we were at the beginning of a long Fourth of July weekend. I looked up Darvon and learned that it lasts in the urine for only two to four days, so I was in the clear. Something is better than nothing, and I had been feeling unusually blue, so I helped myself to about six pills, three times the normal dose. I didn't get high at all from these pills, felt profoundly guilty, thought of this as a wasted effort, and put them entirely out of my mind.

The next day, I had to pull over the car on the way back from a trip to Drumlin Farm with my twin brother, Martin, and the kids, because I was vomiting. I didn't connect the Darvon with the vomiting, because the pills had no effect on me at the time.

*　　*　　*

Two weeks later, midsummer 2007, I was enjoying a rare vacation with Annie and Milo, along with my parents, at the home of an old family friend in Nantucket. This friend was a Yale alum, a businessman, with dark hair and a dark mustache, tall and very decorous, but relaxed and inviting all the same.

The first thing Milo, now aged six, did upon arriving was, inexplicably, toss one of his sandals over the fence and nail, dead-on, our friend's gigantic trophy horseshoe-crab shell, which was prominently displayed on the outer wall of the cottage. Watching it fall down and shatter into a million little pieces, we collectively gasped. Our host visibly girded himself for a long three days of mayhem.

Once we all recovered from the embarrassment and trauma of this, and were finished apologizing profusely, we started enjoying walks along the cobblestoned roads, walks to the beach, walks on the piers looking at the fancy boats, and trips to the playgrounds, eating ice cream, and people watching.

On our first afternoon, back from the beaches, we were all relaxing in our friend's courtyard, eating hors d'oeuvres, when I received a phone call from an unknown number. The voice on the line was incredibly serious. "Hello, this is Dr. Fox. I'm an associate director of SHP, filling in for Dr. Stern. Is this Dr. Grinspoon?" *Oh shit.* This wasn't going to be good. I excused myself and went upstairs.

"Doctor Grinspoon, is there anything you would like to tell us?"
"Umm, like what?"
"Is there anything you would like to disclose?"
"Umm, like what?"

I had no idea what he was getting at.
Dr. Fox continued:

"Are there any prescriptions that you are on, that we don't know about?"
"Umm, like what?"

Is he talking about the Darvon? That's not even possible. That was two weeks ago. There's no way I would incriminate myself.

"I'm sorry to inform you of this, but one of your drug tests came back positive for propoxyphene (Darvon). We need you to come in right away, repeat the test, and sign a new monitoring contract. We are obligated to report this to the medical board."

My only response on the phone for several minutes was to say "Excuse me" in order to buy enough time to figure out which suicide plan to implement. I gave it the old college try: "That's not possible. I didn't take anything. Are you sure they didn't switch the samples?" I went on to protest my innocence for about ten minutes. As the conversation progressed, I increasingly wanted to believe what I was saying, though in the back of my mind I remembered the Darvon. *This can't be happening.*

"Our system is as close to airtight as it gets. Can you come in Monday for a test?"

"Umm, no, I'm in Nantucket with my family on vacation, and the soonest test I can get is on Wednesday, when I'm back in town. I know that sounds dubious but it's true. I can send you the itinerary when I get back in town."

"Wednesday it is. Take care of yourself. Be careful. Go to a meeting. Really, I wish you the best."

My next step was to call my primary care doctor. I explained what had happened, as well as what was certain to result as a consequence. I asked him for a prescription for just a few pills of Darvon, to look like I'd had a valid prescription. I could then hope that SHP wouldn't notice that the prescription would have been written after the test result came back. My PCP said, "Peter, I feel for what you are going through, but I can't do that."

The next thing I did was freak out. This was a silent, internalized freak-out, because I was on an island vacation with my parents, whom I didn't want to disappoint or discuss this with, and with my two small children, who needed me to be emotionally stable. I was forced to act as if everything was OK, which was even more emotionally draining than receiving the cataclysmic news in the first place.

Desperate for someone to talk to about this, and to help me process, I called my girlfriend, Sarah, who was a good listener, and a kind soul. I couldn't tell her that I tested positive for Darvon or she'd know I stole it from her mom, which would, if possible, compound my problems and put a damper on our young relationship. I made up a chemical name and told her that I tested positive for "glucothionide."

I felt sick with myself for lying, first to SHP and then to Sarah, but desperate times called for desperate measures.

I was walking on the beach, one eye on the children at the playground, one ear affixed to my cell phone. Sarah returned me to temporary sanity: "Peter, you've been in this position before, and you've always managed to land on your feet. This will blow over." True, but I was lying to everyone and still taking drugs. How long could this really go on?

Internally, I was preoccupied by two equally painful visions. The first was of sitting down with the medical board and explaining why I had a positive test just when they were getting around to thinking about giving me the green light to go back to work. The second was having to tell H. about this positive test. Both of these visions would come to pass, and they made Dante's Inferno look like an air-conditioned vacation retreat with free drinks (and free refills).

This positive test was also a significant blow in the ideological war to characterize our divorce. It bolstered H.'s attempts to define my addiction as the causative factor in our demise. I had only two weeks left with Maria, and I was worried that she would go ballistic, and that this positive test would land me back in front of the judge again. What was I thinking?

Our friend's house in Nantucket was quaint, with interesting architecture and a deep, old-fashioned, New England charm. It was almost three hundred years old, and filled with antique furniture. The plumbing was as old as the rest of the house. On the last morning of our vacation, having stress-eaten enough food for a small African tribe on the previous day, I plugged the toilet.

I couldn't in good conscience leave this mess for our dignified and gracious host to deal with. After all, we had already pulverized his prize horseshoe-crab shell and trampled on the rest of his house. I scoured the upper floors and the attic and eventually found an antiquated and barely operable toilet plunger from circa the seventeenth century. For the next twenty minutes, I was plunging and in turn viciously stabbing at the blockage with a primitive spear I fashioned by untangling a coat hanger.

My vacation ending, soon to face the music with the medical board, and with H., and with SHP, and with Maria, on my knees in front of this intractable toilet with its ancient, narrow, and anemic piping and its stubborn refusal to cooperate, sweating, my arms cramping with exertion, with brown water and bits of toilet paper splashing back up on me, dripping down my forehead, I thought, "Can my life possibly get any worse? This has *got* to change." I had nothing left to look forward to.

All this misery for a few tablets of Darvon, which wasn't even pleasurable and only made me barf. The pain-to-pleasure ratio of drug use, at least for me over the last several years, was worsening by the hour. The occasional timeless nirvana of opiates, Valium, and ganja had long since given way to stunted, guilty highs, anxiety over the testing, and ever-worsening consequences of my misguided judgments.

The noose around my addiction was growing tighter. Each time, a larger percentage of my brain said, "This just isn't worth it." I thought I was done with these poisons after Brittney's wedding. What was it going to take to get me to stop? An overdose? Waking up in the intensive care unit on life support? Am I really going to give up on being a doctor? On being a dad? For what? For these stupid pills that kept sneaking back into my life and poisoning me?

Symbolically enough, I think it was at the exact moment that I unplugged this toilet, in August of 2007, with a cathartic flush, that my addiction ended. There have been no slips since. It was as if I saw my addiction washing away from me. I had lost almost everything to this addiction. At the rate it was going, there soon wouldn't be anything left. I was getting further from working, and further from my kids. I felt I was letting Danny down by not living up to life's potential.

By self-destructing again and again, I was abandoning my ideals and my higher power. I couldn't continue to be so selfish and to live with myself. This is not a life worth living. At least, not for me. In many ways, it was my worst-case scenario. Alone, miserable, powerless, and disconnected. Unproductive. Ashamed. It was a long and growing list.

At this moment, for whatever reason, I was able to see with clarity that my life had become a game of not getting caught, rather than truly embracing what most mattered to me. I couldn't let my family down again, especially Annie and Milo. I had an almost physical sensation of a new resolve forming within me, a resolve that would come to be tested, again and again, in a myriad of ways, but that would not bend.

In response to this positive test for Darvon, I met again with the medical board, once again down in their airless, fluorescent basement. They added an aggressive stipulation to my already-suspended medical license. This new clause prohibited me from prescribing any controlled substance through the first year of any potential future return to medicine. I would have to have another doctor cosign on my prescriptions for anything but penicillin and Lipitor.

This limitation on my prescribing made me an even less attractive job applicant. If a patient developed sciatica or broke a bone, I would have to ask a colleague to prescribe a painkiller for them. This would give the other providers in the practice not just the hassle but also the legal liability of prescribing extra pain medication.

After this meeting with the board, Solomon, who had shared my fear that I'd be banished from medicine outright, said, "This was a home run; no, actually, it was a triple, and I was expecting to strike out." I *still* had a chance to return to medicine, if I could keep clean. To this day, I'm not sure why the board, and SHP, gave me so many second and third chances.

This positive test had ramifications for my coparenting, such as it was, with H. To start, I couldn't drive the kids for a month. Our divorce agreement states:

> The Husband shall promptly inform the Wife in writing (i.e. e-mail, fax, etc.) and orally of any dilute or positive drug test results or of any change to the Society to Help Physicians ("SHP") protocol or contract. If a test result is an unexplained positive one...his overnight parenting shall be supervised by a family member, and the Husband's driving the children during his visitation shall be suspended until he completes and provides negative drug test results for a thirty (30) day period.

The "supervised by a family member" was covered because I was living with my parents. It must have looked ridiculous, to have a graying woman in her late seventies chauffeuring her forty-year-old child and two grandchildren to birthday parties and playdates. It must have been stressful on my mom, who wanted to enjoy retirement and to believe her son was on the mend.

During this time, miraculously, despite the Vicodin at Brittney's wedding, and the Darvon, I was making slow and halting progress toward a potential return to work.

I looked better. My eyes were no longer glazed over or bloodshot. I had lost much of the hand shaking that had plagued me since stopping Klonapin at Tannenberg two years earlier. My sleep was better, less drugged, and I was starting to remember my dreams again.

I was exercising, hard, every day. A healthy nirvana. Nobody begrudges endorphins.

When we were married, H. had prohibited me from walking out of the house without a shirt, because of my gut. Not one to mince words, she said, "You are too fat to walk around without a shirt. Put on a shirt right now, or get back in the house."

Later, when I dropped off the kids, she complained bitterly, "We're separated and now you're all buff."

My thoughts were quicker and more fluid every day. There was less of a dull haze hovering between my brain and the outside world. I was starting to feel centered and focused again after ten years of fogginess. The different parts of my psyche were recoalescing.

There were two weeks left on my two years of probation when Maria found out about the positive results for Darvon, which is partly why I was so profoundly stressed in Nantucket. I had come too far to have this ripped away. I could still get into major trouble, all for stupid, fucking Darvon, a non-high that made me barf, a pink pill that reached from the grave of my addiction and tried to drag me back to that hellish place.

Instead of surrendering me and my broiled tuckus, on a platter, to the judge for execution, Maria let this slide. She briefly wished me well and submerged back into her basement den of iniquity. After all that fuss and stress, the criminal charges automatically expired, not with a bang but a whimper.

Why did Maria let me go? She must have decided that I was going to do all right, at least compared with her other clients. Or maybe she thought I didn't really belong there in the first place. I suppose, after two years, she was tired of dealing with me. During our meetings, her stern reticence made me nervous and brought out my chitchat. She mentioned several times that I was giving her a headache. I drove up her Excedrin bills.

Being finally free of Maria was a momentous and emotionally laden event for me, but there was no celebration, no party, no balloons, no handshakes or backslaps, certainly no champagne. It's hard to celebrate the absence of a negative. We celebrate positives such as birth or marriage. No one celebrates not getting hit by a bus. Or not having criminal charges filed against you. Over the phone, my brother David said, "You're getting there. Don't give up on this. God and the universe are one!"

Even though they were dismissed, the criminal complaints against me will always be public record, like a scar that never entirely fades. The court papers implicating me will forever be moldering in the West Roxbury courthouse. Prospective employers who did their homework would know about them.

At least I was free of the possibility of criminal convictions, fines, and jail time. I no longer had to sit in that basement with those drugged-out thugs anymore. My kneecaps breathed a sigh of relief, now that they were safe from stapler-hurling counselors. So did my fingers, knowing they wouldn't be assaulted and bruised again by Rufus and his ilk.

To this day, I'm still not sure if I could pass the CORI (Criminal Offender Record Information) check needed to accompany my children on field trips or to volunteer at school events. Purportedly, all cases heard before a judge in Massachusetts show up, though I'm not sure if this record persists indefinitely when the charges are dropped.

Solomon said enough time had finally passed, and that I could start reaching out to potential employers about an eventual return to work. I had to disclose two things up front: I wouldn't be sure if and when I'd get my license back, and I was prohibited from prescribing controlled substances for at least a year after starting.

The best I could say was that I likely would enter a probation agreement with the board, which probably would result in their approval to return to work within the next year. In other words, a hard pill to swallow for a prospective employer looking for certainty and stability, even if they were brave (or foolish) enough to take a chance on an addict.

Solomon said that even a provisional commitment from a reputable employer would help nudge the board to give their consent, because it would help them envision me in a secure employment situation that could be closely monitored. He again acknowledged this catch-22, that a job would help me get my license but that my license would help me get a job. He conceded that this would require some finesse and some luck.

The process of looking for a job without a medical license, with no certain timeline for its return, with criminal charges on file, not having worked for several years, seemed like a hard sell. This process promised to be about as uplifting and successful as my recent Internet dating experiences, trying to sell myself as a suitable mate while living with my parents and being possibly unemployable.

The first job I interviewed for was at Newton-Wellesley Hospital. This hospital is near my childhood home, and it is where we had brought my friend Will when he freaked out on acid, when we were experimenting with it in high school. In fact, the last time I had been in this hospital, I was standing next to Will's bed, with him tethered down in four-point restraints and with his parents staring reprovingly at me, as if it were *my idea* to drop acid.

This hospital had a reputation for being second-rate, compared to the downtown academic hospitals, as I was growing up. Certainly my dad, ensconced in Harvard, put it down at every opportunity. I thought I should apply there to test the water, because beggars can't be choosers, and it wouldn't hurt me to slum it for a while at the local hospital until I was back on my feet.

After I had waited awhile in a comfortable lobby, the chief of service came in to speak with me. He was an elderly surgeon who was affable and direct, if somewhat condescending. He listened patiently to my story and my petition to be considered for employment. He replied, "You seem like a nice guy, and I appreciate your honesty. You've got excellent training, and I'd like to help you. But the doctors here are conservative. They aren't open-minded. They would never go for this. We would like to think of ourselves as the type of people who would hire someone like you, but we just aren't. Best of luck in your search." I was dismissed.

Shot down by the second-rate hospital of my childhood! This didn't bode so well.

Seeking to plant my petition in more sympathetic soil, I returned to my roots and applied at Boston Medical Center, where, ten years earlier, I had graduated as their "star" student. Maybe they still needed doctors to take care of the impoverished ghetto dwellers and immigrants, and would welcome my damaged candidacy.

The medicine department at Boston Medical was progressive and enlightened about addiction. The chief of service was a substance abuse specialist who had been one of my mentors. They knew me and empathized with what had happened to me. They understood that addiction can happen to anyone, especially doctors, that it is a disease, and that it can be successfully treated.

After several rounds of intensive interviewing, they concluded that I was still the same Peter as before, who would work hard and care about patients. They offered me a dream job as part of their primary care team, working in their front-line clinics. They invited me to work with, and mentor, any other physicians that encountered addiction.

As a condition of employment, they insisted that I continue to be monitored by SHP, not only for a few more years but until the end of time. I had no choice but to agree. They were also concerned about a scenario where I might pressure junior doctors who were under my supervision for prescriptions, using my power over them to extract favors. They created a questionnaire for the junior doctors about my interactions with them, asking them if "Dr. Grinspoon at any time asked or pressured you to write or fill a prescription for him."

As Boston Medical is a public hospital, my job offer was contingent on approval by the various hospital supervisory committees, which took months. Once I had cleared these hurdles and had a definitive job offer, then I could petition the board to activate my license.

I was elated. After all of the turmoil, I had finally received a job offer, even if it was conditional. I didn't for a moment suspect that I would be rejected in committee. Returning to work would wipe away at least a small part of my shame, and be a step toward getting my life back. I would recover a few crumbs of my depleted dignity. It also symbolized my healing process. I was getting there.

I passed through several of these committees unanimously. The doctors all gave me the thumbs-up and seemed to believe in giving people second chances. All that stood in my way was one last committee, which included several laypeople in addition to physicians, as a way to ensure community representation for this public hospital.

On this final vote, every single doctor sided with me, and every single one of the laypeople voted against me. A tie vote meant no, with no mechanism to appeal. After four months of waiting, and hoping, and planning, and fantasizing, and shaving, and starting to dig out nicer clothes to wear, and starting to feel better about myself, I was back to square one.

When I next spoke with the medical director at the Shattuck Hospital, that sad hospital of last resort on the fringes of society, where I attended my first Narcotics Anonymous meetings, he said, "I've heard you are a remarkable individual, but we don't have any current openings." Not even this shabby deathtrap of last hope would hire me.

As 2007 turned into 2008, I was still applying for jobs, though I wasn't entirely discouraged because I had started getting noticeably better vibes from prospective employers. There was a worsening shortage of primary care doctors, which, with my training and pedigree, made me somewhat of an attractive commodity, if one could only ignore the criminal charges and suspended medical license.

With repetition and practice, I came across as less glib, nervous, and guilty when describing my predicament. Each day, I continued to be monitored by SHP, which added a level of comfort and allowed me to build up a solid track record of sobriety.

As the clock ticked, I was further away from the criminal charges, and further into documented recovery, but I was also further away from having practiced medicine. It was getting on three years.

I was concerned about all of the little things I might be forgetting, the subtle curve on a cardiogram that could suggest a heart attack, or the hard-to-recognize "slapped cheek" rash that suggests parvovirus. Clinical instincts are not things you can easily relearn from a book, and I feared that mine were getting pretty rusty.

Some doctors who have been out of work are required by the board to attend months of skills retraining, at great cost. This was particularly true for surgeons, who needed to regain their delicate precision touch before returning to the operating room. I was desperate to get back to work before any of this became necessary.

My next big job interview was at a large community health center located in a down-and-out part of Boston. This clinic was located just over the Tobin Bridge from the gleaming spires of its mother ship, Man's Greatest Hospital (MGH). I was asked for money twice in the parking lot of this health center, by racially diverse and multicultural beggars, as I walked from my car to the interview.

The patients here were predominantly Hispanic, from Latin America. They were poor and often didn't speak English. Some of them were illiterate. The waiting room also hosted patients from Ethiopia, Serbia, Sierra Leone, and Haiti. It reminded me of Boston City Hospital, where I had so many adrenaline-filled adventures in medical school, but where my life had started to derail.

My first job out of residency involved caring for the well-to-do and entitled, the "worried well," for whom pimples and wrinkles could be absolute emergencies. My second job at the Faulkner featured a patient population that was predominantly working-class. If I were to be hired at this health center, with its impoverished patients, the general trajectory of my career from doctor to the rich to doctor of the destitute would continue. At this rate, in my next job I'd be working in a prison, or in a slum in India, or possibly with Paul Farmer in Haiti (which would be an honor).

After a grueling sequence of interviews over two weeks, eighteen of the twenty doctors voted to hire me, which was enough. Luckily, they didn't test my Spanish, which was mediocre at best; my comically gringo accent alone would have lost me the job. To this day, staff members sob in laughter when they hear my accent, even in front of patients, which makes me self-conscious.

This health center made me a job offer as a part-time primary care doctor, which was solid enough to present to the medical board. When I received this news, I was euphoric. I called Martin. "MGH offered me a job. What are they thinking? It's MGH!" I couldn't wait to start. Not only did I now have a job offer, but it was an excellent job, doing important work, with people who needed the help. I promised myself that if this came through, I wouldn't screw it up.

There were two related obstacles: I didn't have a medical license and, somehow, I had managed to flunk another drug test.

After years of cheating the system, gaming the tests, drinking water, diluting the samples, dragging my feet, I had finally, with the help of SHP and my support community, and the threat of the board, become entirely free of drugs. The Darvon, which I symbolically flushed down the toilet in 2007, had been the last straw, and it had been smooth sailing ever since.

And *now*, as I'm knocking on the door of my dream job, I flunk a test. Was this karmic revenge for being such a sneak over the last few years? Karmic revenge for being such a liar? God's sense of irony?

I tested positive for Oxazepam, a mild sleeping pill, Valium light, in both February and May of 2008.

Drug addicts are almost always guilty until proven innocent, but not even the staff at SHP, who seemed to be clinically paranoid about relapses, were convinced that I had relapsed. During an emergency meeting, Dr. Stern, who looked visibly puzzled, said, "You've had a pair of positive tests but there is no other information to suggest a relapse."

His assessment was that I hadn't relapsed, but that there might have been some minor slippage. To be sure, he ordered extra urine and hair tests, and required me to attend more frequent meetings. He continued with his customary bluntness, "You can't work until this stops happening. I'm concerned that you are trying to sabotage your own return to work. Every time you have a positive test, or a dilute, it leads to a lower level of trust at SHP. There is very little trust left."

Miraculously, the MGH clinic stood by their job offer, despite these positive tests. They must have sniffed that I hadn't relapsed as well. They ignored the fact that H. kept serving me nasty-looking court documents at the clinic, even before I had started working there. These documents were liberally peppered with "drug addict" and "lied to the judge." The secretaries had to sign for them and store them for me.

I remain amazed at the faith the staff at the clinic put in me, and the way they stuck with me through all of this negative press and uncertainty. Part of it might have been that they needed to replace the two male doctors who had just been sacked, one for making sexually charged comments to female staff members, and the other for making too many home visits to his young, nubile, female patients. (For these home visits, he didn't get in any trouble with the medical board, which supports my theory that what the board finds out about and punishes is completely arbitrary.)

The unit chief, Dr. Z., is a few years younger than me. He is thin, of medium height, with thick, wavy, graying brown hair. He dresses in a dapper, even foppish manner. He is known to be fair in disputes and to always be joking. If you complain or whine to him about something trivial, he might smile and say, "I'll put that on the top of the list of things I don't care about." He is an outstanding doctor, even if he does say to me "Shut the fuck up, I'm trying to work" about four times a day. (We share an office, so he's the unfortunate person I bounce ideas off of.)

He was concerned enough about the positive tests for Oxazepam to ask me to come in and explain the results in person. He sat me down, shut the door, looked me in the eye, and said, "Did you take Oxazepam?" to which, for once, I could answer with entire honesty in the negative. He didn't revoke the job offer.

The medical board still needed to give me the green light and, if I learned anything at all from Solomon and from the last three years, it was that the Massachusetts Medical Board is *not* predictable. I needed them to give their approval rapidly, because I couldn't expect this job offer to remain open indefinitely.

The job offer was made to me in August of 2008. Solomon managed to get my case in front of the board on November 19, 2008. I waited in the lobby nervously for hours, making small talk with one of Solomon's junior associates, who had accompanied me.

After a few hours, I was at the end of my rope. I was about to give up, concede and surrender, and go home in defeat. I kept repeating Nate's words to fortify myself: "It ain't over 'til you are six feet under and they're shoveling dirt on your face." I was sure they were going to shoot me down. I had screwed up too many times to count, and they weren't known to be that forgiving.

After an eternity of waiting, a kind, portly, middle-aged woman with brown hair and a brown business suit sauntered out, ambled over to where I was sitting, gave me a warm smile, grabbed my hand, and said, "Congratulations, Dr. Grinspoon, the board has approved your petition to return to work. Great job on your recovery. Good luck."

Solomon's associate gave me a congratulatory hug. Hugs from attorneys are done in a formal and anatomically correct manner; they are polite and they don't cross any boundaries, but somehow they fail to convey warmth or human connection. At that point, in my elation, I would have hugged a porcupine or a python.

Six days later, on November 25, after a three-and-a-half-year hiatus, I was back at work, about to see my first patient. There were heavy restrictions in place. I had several years left on my SHP contract and would continue my drug testing and my support group meetings. I had a work site monitor who kept tabs on me. I couldn't prescribe anything stronger than penicillin without asking a colleague, or one of the nurse practitioners, to physically write the prescription. I was on a provisional and temporary credentialing status with all of the insurance companies. I was still blackballed by the American Board of Internal Medicine.

But I didn't care. I was so excited to be back at work, all of these details seemed trivial. As time ticked on, the restrictions would fall by the wayside.

On my first day back, I closed the door to my small windowless office at the health center in order to have a few moments to gather myself. I briefly lamented the loss of my previous office at the Faulkner, with its spaciousness and its spectacular vista over the Arnold Arboretum. I hadn't necessarily come down in the world, being at the almighty MGH, but my office certainly wasn't as swank.

I struggled to learn the new electronic medical record system, which was an improvement over the dark ages of paper charts, where, more often than not, I couldn't read handwriting or find reports. If I accidentally dropped a paper chart, it could take hours to put Humpty together again.

While I was anxiously waiting for the medical assistant to announce my first patient, I accidentally deleted my preliminary note, as a consequence of too much nervous fiddling. I was trying to look busy but, without any patients, I didn't have much to do.

My plump, Latina medical assistant announced, in her sing-song Hispanic voice, "Dr. Greeenspoon, dere is a patient waiting for you in de exam room." Showtime.

Now that it was finally time to enter the exam room, I was flooded with contradictory emotions. In some ways, this process felt automatic, like riding a bike. I had performed this act tens of thousands of times during my first five years of practice, and part of my brain was extremely confident.

The process also felt deliberate and self-conscious, because I had obsessed and fantasized about it for more than three years. It felt like asking someone to dance after being married to someone else for ten years. I would feel awkward and uncomfortable until the music started up.

The cocky, addictive part of me felt like a marauding, medical Caesar, who had defied all of the odds and who couldn't be kept down, even by the Fates themselves, or the board, or the police, or the DEA, or Maria. Can't touch this. Another part of me felt like a neophyte medical student, stammering, stuttering, forcing myself to pretend that I was in command of what I was doing.

Overall, I was humbled and genuinely grateful to have another chance.

Walking into this exam room, I was walking straight into all of the prejudices about physicians and addiction that I had faced down in the last four years, and which I was still highly insecure about. Had this patient Googled me? Had they read the press releases about my drug charges? Were they seeing me only because the other doctors were busy, or because it was an underserved community?

I didn't yet know that many of my new patients couldn't read, didn't speak English, and were too poor and downtrodden to care about whether their doctor did drugs in the past. They have their own preoccupations.

I remembered Dr. Stern telling me that when I went back, I had to hold my head high. I could hear my neck muscles creaking as I forced my line of sight up from the floor to a level plane.

"Hi, Candice, I'm Dr. Grinspoon, your new doctor. How can I help you today?"

Stressful as this transition was, I was ecstatic to be back in the saddle again, and I knew that if I kept, as Dr. Stern suggested, "putting one foot in front of the other," sooner or later I would fall back into a routine, and providing primary care would once again become second nature. I continued to dust off my responses to different scenarios: earwax, foot pain, high sugar, back spasm, constipation, hives.

My patients at this practice were challenging. I thought that one Spanish-speaking gentleman was saying to me, "I fell off a donkey fourteen years ago and a stick rammed into my butt, and now it's hurting." Fearing that I had vastly overestimated my Spanish language skills, I rushed to get my medical assistant to translate. After conferring with the patient, she said, "He fell off a donkey fourteen years ago and a stick stuck into his bottom, and now it hurts." We never learned about distant donkey-butt injuries in medical school. The Distant Ass Butt Syndrome.

I deliberately resisted the urge to skulk around in the shadows of the hospitals and to avoid my former colleagues and acquaintances. Sure, some of them would look down their noses at me. Some of them would never see me as separate from my drug use and my recently suspended license. I could perceive this when I spoke to them, a subtly self-righteous attitude that betrayed them despite their otherwise polite conversation.

These prejudices were part of the daily obstacles I faced, along with stacks of lab results to dictate and piles of papers to sign off on. I suspected that they would fade over time.

It helped tremendously that all of the docs I worked with at my health center knew about my addiction and were supportive. At least the eighteen of twenty who voted to hire me were. This was a core group who didn't judge me. As inner-city primary care docs, they were addiction savvy, so they knew the long odds for most addicts, and were impressed with what I had overcome.

My colleagues were gracious about signing the narcotic prescriptions for my patients, which I was prohibited from doing. They were good-natured about acting as monitors and sending in the paperwork for my SHP contract.

I did my best not to wear out my welcome, or to cause them to suspect me and question their decision. I made extra sure not to appear sleepy or confused at work, though most primary care doctors look sleepy and confused on a good day. Having chronic hay fever didn't help my campaign to avoid bloodshot eyes. I was most worried that I would be the first to be suspected if any drugs or prescriptions went missing from the office.

I remained self-conscious about the secretarial and support staff finding out about my addiction and the criminal charges. I didn't want the entire staff gossiping about it, or not trusting me because of scary preconceived notions of drug addicts.

One patient, during her first visit with me, announced to the front desk, "Look what I found online. Who's this new doctor you want me to see? His license was suspended. Did you know there were criminal charges? For drug use!" She's actually one of my favorite patients, to this day, just a little disinhibited. She said she was nervous about meeting her new doctor, and was only making conversation.

As days became weeks, months, and then years, the restrictions on my practice were slowly eased, expired, or were eventually phased out, and the daily reminders of my addiction started to fade into the background. It was like gluing back the discarded layers of an onion to create something that resembles the original, though with small fault lines where the layers had been ripped off. In some places, the glue makes the finished product even stronger than the original, while in others there will always remain damaged tissue and vulnerabilities.

I had no more problems with dilute or positive drug tests. I never entirely lost my fear of the false-positive test result due to a switched sample or a lab error. The false positive early in 2008 for Oxazepam had almost derailed my return to work.

I was exposed to healthy doses of temptation shortly after going back into practice. Medicine is a land of unique opportunity for a drug addict. There are pills galore in every doctor's office. Even in our office, which, as a policy, doesn't cravenly accept drug company handouts, there is unlimited access.

As part of a recent push in patient safety, primary care docs are being asked to reconcile the medications a patient is taking at home with their computerized medication list. This ensures that patients are taking what we think they are taking, especially after a hospitalization, when many different cooks enter the mix and muck around with the meds.

Often, patients are discharged home and end up taking duplicate medications, which is potentially toxic. It's easy to take Lipitor and atorvastatin if you don't know they are the same medicine.

The only practical way to reconcile the meds is for the patients to bring all of their bottles of medication with them to their primary care visit, so that we can go through the bottles one by one, update the list in the computer, and eliminate extra bottles of medications. We can then give the patients an updated list, which we know is accurate, and they return home with bottles that correspond to this list. This practice clearly saves lives and prevents readmission to the hospital.

We dispose of superfluous medications that would otherwise clutter medicine cabinets and invite medical mistakes. Technically, these extraneous medications are supposed to be incinerated rather than flushed, so they don't enter the water supply and get the birds and fish too stoned. In reality, because of the time pressure we are under, we just dump them into the trash. No one supervises this in the clinic setting.

The earlier, drugged-out version of me would have circled back to retrieve these medications from the trash as soon as the patient left the room. I then would have transferred the pills to a different bottle in my bag, marked ALLEGRA or ZANTAC. I'd dispose of the original bottle, so there would be no chain of evidence connecting these pills to their original source. This was practically foolproof because, short of a forensic laboratory, it is impossible to tell which pills are which.

A few times since being back at work, hearing the siren song of the pills, entranced, I started to circle back toward the exam rooms with freshly discarded pills waiting in the trash cans. I stopped myself with a quick reminder that I didn't want to go down that path, or even anywhere near that path. That path led me directly back to Maria's basement and the judge, and it led me away from Annie and Milo. I had already spent enough time being broiled by the medical board.

Over time, these pills sing to me less, but if I listen carefully, they still quietly beckon.

Almost immediately upon returning to work, I stumbled into a dilemma involving my care for drug-addicted patients. Many of these patients were young opiate addicts who could have been myself sitting there, a few years earlier, something the cat dragged in, flushed, fidgety, sweaty, with red and defiant eyes.

I could see the walls surrounding them, walls of false bravado constructed from denial and need. Most of them were braced to pit whatever wits they had remaining against this doctor, in order to leave the visit with a scrip for painkillers in hand. I was a necessary means to either a euphoric or a lucrative end. With effort, they usually managed some elemental politeness, but tended to be pushy and goal-directed.

Some of these patients needed papers signed for their probation officers, saying that, as far as I was aware, they had stayed out of drug-related trouble. Some needed pee tests. Others were just released from jail, having served time for drug-related offenses or for other crimes, such as bank robbery, to support their habits.

Many of my patients were polyaddicted, most commonly to opiates and cocaine. Some were sincerely trying to get clean.

I never understood why inmates are released from incarceration with only a one-week supply of their psych meds, and no organized follow-up. They are told to "find a doctor." It's almost impossible to get into even your primary care doctor's office within a few weeks, let alone get specialized psychiatric care. Most of these patients seemed to end up off their meds and relapsing on the drugs that got them in trouble in the first place.

The treatment success in prison seemed even worse than Maria's basement, and we inner-city primary care docs were expected to pick up the pieces. As I was well aware, these patients didn't have much to look forward to. It's all but impossible to land a good job with a criminal record, and it's difficult to stay sober if your psych meds abruptly run out and your addiction is untreated.

During my first few visits with my addicted patients, I realized that there was no fundamental difference between them and me. The trappings of our lives were different, but addicts are addicts, with the same symptoms and vulnerabilities. Our brain disease was identical. These addicts were people I could have attended Narcotics Anonymous meetings with, or they might have been in my therapy group in Maria's basement. They were my brothers-in-arms.

Once I realized our sameness, I very much wanted to connect with them addict-to-addict, as I had been doing all along with members of the recovery community in all other walks of my life, such as my recovery meetings. All my instincts wanted me to say, "Hi, I'm Peter, and I'm an addict too. What's your story? Let's go to a meeting." This is what I might say if I happened to bump into the exact same person at a Narcotics Anonymous meeting.

I couldn't bring myself to do this. I wondered to myself, "Why should my personal response to these addicts vary so much from my response to other addicts, according to the setting?"

I came to realize that the collaborative, brotherly-love approach utilized in recovery didn't even remotely fit the context of my role as their doctor. I wasn't Peter the addict, no last names, we're all equal and in this together. I was Dr. Grinspoon, whom you have to listen to if you want to get better, appease your probation officer, or receive a prescription. I was an authority figure, part of the machinery that was keeping them in line. This isn't to say that I wasn't nice to them, just that there was an insuperable distance between us.

To be one of the addicts, one of the gang, would have demolished the necessary authority to heal, and would have made it impossible to act in the role of a doctor. The doctor-patient relationship comes with a ready-made barrier, which I unconsciously hid behind. At times I felt as if I were acting with hypocrisy toward my fellow addicts, like I was some nouveau riche ditching my humble old friends for better ones.

Dr. Stern, my soothsayer, had, as usual, foreseen a future in which I had to confront this issue. He had suggested, "Tell people about your addiction if you think it would help." I didn't think to ask him "Help who, me or the other addicts?" I think he meant if it would help the situation in general.

I decided that "coming out" at work wouldn't be helpful to these patients or to myself. They wouldn't relate to or learn from my experiences, because they lived on a different planet. Your typical teenage gang member wouldn't sympathize with, for example, my complaints of a delayed board certification in internal medicine. They want a fix, or to get into treatment right away. They couldn't afford rehab, and didn't have anything as salient as a medical license to lose. They didn't have the 80 percent success rate that doctors do. Most of them would relapse.

I didn't want patients to seek me out for favors, under the mistaken belief that I was still on the wrong side of the line. I'd be seen as one of the "drug doctors," and patients might think they could get easy scrips from me.

For the sake of self-preservation, I needed to stay away from, rather than attract, the criminal element. I didn't want to be tempted back toward that lifestyle. I am happy to take care of my share of these patients, but why advertise for more? If anything, I would overidentify with them. With my potential to screw up boundaries wherever drugs are involved, who knows what I could get myself into?

Better to keep my druggie past separate from my current medical career, though there is a limit to how separate they can be within the confines of one personality. As the writer André Gide wrote, "We are the sum total of our experiences." The experiences I've had, the good as well as the ugly, deeply influence the medical care I provide, especially to other addicts.

I was tending to a patient whose care I assumed from another doc who had just left our practice. Before meeting him, my radar was on maximum alert, because he was one of those patients who are on a gigantic dose of the painkiller methadone to treat an ill-defined pain syndrome. No broken bone on X-ray. No arthritis or cancer. He had only his vehement complaints of back pain as evidence. He had a criminal history and a drug history, which further elevated my suspicion.

F.C. came into my office accompanied by his long-standing girlfriend and, as it turned out, drug buddy. F.C. was dressed in dungarees and a flannel shirt, and had graying hair, a slight paunch, and a pleasant demeanor that turned on a dime when you crossed him, into pure viciousness. He limped into my office.

I hadn't yet had an opportunity to confirm if he really had a limp by my time-tested method of following him out of the office into the parking lot and seeing if he still limped when no one was watching. I've caught several patients by doing this. With F.C., I attempted some pleasantries, but he got right down to business.

"*Doc, listen to me carefully. I'm in pain. The 110 milligrams of methadone isn't cutting it. I need to go up to 120.*"

"As your new doctor, we need to discuss your general health history before we talk about anything in particular, especially prescriptions for narcotics."

"*Doc, you aren't* listening. *I asked you to listen. My back is hurting bad. I need some more medication. I need a bigger dose of methadone.*"

"I don't feel comfortable prescribing methadone at all. I hardly ever prescribe this. It should be done by a pain specialist, especially given the large dose you are on. It needs to be monitored by specialists. We don't use this for pain anymore. We have other ways to treat pain. Such as physical therapy, or a steroid injection. Methadone is especially dangerous, given that you've used drugs before."

(Emitting steam and sparks) "I'm in recovery. I haven't done any drugs in five years. We go to recovery meetings five nights a week. (Pointing at me) Don't you go saying I'm on drugs. I can't take this pain anymore. Read my chart. Nothing else worked. I need to go up to 120."

"You should consider a methadone clinic for this. I'll continue your current dosage today, because that's what we've been giving you, and it's what you expected from Dr. Walsh, so you don't withdraw. I have to think about this and consult with some pain and addiction specialists. Here's your scrip. You need to provide me with a urine specimen on the way out."

I needed the urine specimen to make sure he wasn't taking anything else on the side, like cocaine or meth, which might interact with the methadone and cause his heart to stop. I also needed to check that he was indeed taking this methadone and not selling his prescription. His drug screen should show some methadone in it, but nothing else.

Because F.C. and his girlfriend had so sincerely touted the quality of their recovery, and because I could imagine sitting next to them at a Narcotics Anonymous meeting, I felt vaguely guilty policing them so aggressively and in such an intrusive manner with this drug screen. But better safe than sorry.

Prescription in hand, though not at the dose he wanted, F.C. stormed out of my office. Twenty minutes later, my medical assistant came in. "Mr. C. didn't leave a urine specimen. He had to leave immediately to visit his daughter in the emergency room. She just had a car accident." Sorry, we'll have to get that pesky little urine test another time.

A car accident? When? It didn't sound right. Wouldn't he have mentioned the accident to me during our visit? Did his daughter have the accident in the ten seconds that elapsed between leaving my office and walking to the front desk? What are the chances this would occur during our first visit?

Scanning the chart, I saw that he hadn't provided any recent drug screens. It's easy to grow familiar and let down your guard. I called F.C. and told him that he needed to come in immediately and that, if he ever wanted pain medication from this clinic again, he had better unzip and start peeing pronto. He came back an hour later. The specimen he left was very dilute, which suggests he intentionally drank water the whole time to dilute the specimen. Been there, done that!

Despite these evasive efforts, the specimen came back positive for cocaine and Valium.

When confronted, F.C. looked at me as if I was an unpleasant thing he had to step over. "Doc, I screwed up just that one time. I made a mistake. It was my birthday and someone offered me a few lines of blow at a party. It's the first time I used anything in five years. I can't take this pain anymore. Read my chart. Nothing else worked." Looking straight into my eyes, "Doc, give me another chance. I promise I won't screw up again."

Against my better judgment, and against everything I learned during my drugbatical, I gave him another chance, with a shorter leash, making him come back and see me in person every twenty-eight days to renew his prescription, with drug tests at every visit. Six weeks later, I received a call from a methadone clinic in Boston wishing to touch base with the primary care doctor of one of their new clients. They were as shocked as I was to discover that F.C. was receiving a double dose of methadone, one from each of us.

I cut F.C. off from his pain medications, and he dumped me as his doctor. His name has only come up twice since then. A few months later, he asked me to write a letter attesting that he was too ill to spend any time in jail. His attorney explained that he was caught driving the getaway car during a larceny and preferred to avoid prison. I wanted to know, "Too ill with what? Not-wanting-to-go-to-jail-itis?"

The last contact was when I was called by a psychiatrist trying to evaluate him. She was concerned that he had been fired by his latest pain doctor "for saying racist things" and, additionally, that "he has a gun at home."

Before my drugbatical, I never would have caught on to F.C., and would have kept writing him prescriptions ad infinitum. The methadone scrips might have gone on to this day. Maybe I'd have found a way to get some of his drugs from him, give him some more, skim off the top. Or, once he was busted, I would have written him off as a small-time thug, one of the many who give primary care its variety and flavor, never to be seen again.

Since being addicted myself, and returning to practice, I can still understand him as a small-time thug, but I spend a little bit more time thinking about the person behind the mask. I know that he was just using me for drugs, but part of me wonders who he was before the addiction, and what went wrong. Bad parents? Low IQ? Broken heart? Lead exposure? Untreated depression? Distant Ass Butt Syndrome?

Or are addictions completely independent of personalities and past influences, and is this all just a tug-of-war with a particular group of brain cells that want to be stimulated? It wasn't up to me, with my past and my disease, to judge F.C. as a bad person, rather than someone who needs patient and compassionate care, though it's never fun to be lied to point-blank.

Eighteen months after I returned to work, the DEA accepted my petition and agreed to lift all of the restrictions on my prescribing controlled substances. No more embarrassed and shameful trips to a colleague's office to ask if they could, yet again, sign a prescription for cough syrup with codeine for one of my patients with bronchitis.

One by one, the insurance companies and the HMOs took me off probation and eliminated the need for performance reports from my supervisors. In January 2011, I regained my certification by the American Board of Internal Medicine, after passing their utterly useless and expensive maintenance of certification exam that internists are blackmailed into taking every decade, as a way to ensure that they are sufficiently overworked and burned-out.

The main bureaucracy that remained involved was the medical board. I was still on probation with them. As more time elapsed on my SHP contract, and I had a progressively longer period of demonstrated sobriety, the process of getting the medical board to end my probation should, at some point, have become automatic. I didn't know when that point was, and the board wasn't particularly predictable or internally consistent.

When I was crashing and burning, I was a priority. I had their attention, and they fit me right into their schedule. Now that I was doing well, I was put on the farthest back burner.

Solomon finally secured a commitment from the medical board, but my petition kept slipping from the agenda of meeting after meeting. Into the summer of 2011, I would wait with bated breath each time they met, only to be informed that the meeting was canceled at the last minute because they decided to go on vacation, they didn't have a quorum, or they just didn't have time to address my case.

Because I was employed, there weren't any financial repercussions to this delay, except that I still needed my attorney Solomon on the case, and his fees added up quickly. To me, it was hugely symbolic. The board had been my nemesis all along, the most concrete manifestation of the mess I had made of my life. After all the guilt and the shame I suffered, I was desperate for affirmation by this most conservative and critical of all institutions.

I wanted to achieve the symbolism of having a new wallet card, verifying my medical license, that didn't contain the words "with restrictions" in small black print.

On July 20, 2011, six years after I was compelled by Solomon to sign my (not so) "voluntary agreement not to practice medicine," my probation with the medical board finally ended. Solomon's assistant called me and said, "You're done with the board." No bang, no whimper. No ceremony.

At that moment, I stopped shying away from my former colleagues or cringing at the possibility that someone would Google me and find out what I had done. It didn't matter anymore. The past was truly in my past, more distant every day.

Of course, when you dig a hole as deep as I did, there are dozens of petty bureaucrats in charge of your fate. Some of the insurance companies held on to the restrictions. Their argument was "The successful resolution of board issues does not automatically result in reinstatement." When reapplying for hospital privileges, I will always have a lot of explaining to do, until the end of my career.

The board's approval triggered the end of my SHP contract. No more solemn meetings with Dr. Stern. I had peed in a cup about four hundred times over the last six years, which comes out to about twenty gallons of urine and $18,000 in testing fees. I was now clean, and free.

In early 2012, I was asked by SHP to write up a version of my "story" for their annual report. This led to an invitation to be the keynote speaker at their annual dinner. They must have had faith in my recovery, because they wouldn't want to chance the embarrassment of their speaker relapsing before the speech, especially with their donors, board members, and all of their graduates in the audience.

At Greenpeace, I had done quite a bit of public speaking, but never about myself. It's easier to speak about impersonal topics such as global warming or nuclear power. You just use an angry voice and throw in a lot of rhetoric. When you are preaching to the converted, it's easy to be a successful speaker. Yeah, brother, tell it how it is!

At recovery meetings, I had occasionally told my story, but just to small groups of people, all of whom were themselves addicts and wouldn't be judging me. They didn't even really know who I was, beyond my first name.

Never had I publicly spoken about my addiction. Instead of hiding all aspects of it, as I had been doing for the last eight years, I was going to be *volunteering* the details about it in a public venue. Part of me felt that I was supposed to be putting all of this behind me, certainly not advertising it. I had a debt of gratitude to SHP, so there wasn't much of a choice but to try to give back.

I didn't know how much of my story to share. The audience was partly addicts and partly laypeople and psychiatrists who were affiliated with SHP. Did they want sordid details? I had enough of those to go around. How much should I talk about outsmarting my SHP tests, and skipping meetings? Would this embarrass them? Was it too late to get into trouble? Would they ask me to restart my contract? Would they inform the board?

I've always wanted to be the new Mario Savio, a charismatic public speaker who was so spellbinding that he could literally incite riots, until he was banned from speaking at Berkeley. I was gaining experience at Greenpeace, but then my path through medical school stopped the momentum of my refinement as a public speaker. It's hard to incite riots with educational talks on Pap smears or earwax. "And we must not be afraid to *treat* flat feet, together, with *inserts*!" Thunderous applause. Fist pumping. Time to storm the administration building.

There was a vicious snowstorm on the night of my talk at SHP, which left about forty diehards in attendance. Nervously waiting, I listened to, of all things, a harpist plucking on her instrument. It sounded like a *Star Trek* episode. I expected to see Klingons and Romulans pouring into the room. The sound of the harp put me in a dreamlike state, like the barbiturates used to. I had to keep waking myself up.

I was sitting with my brilliant and even-tempered fiancée, proudly introducing her to my SHP comrades-in-arms, whom I knew well from the recovery meetings. Finally, "...and we now introduce our night's speaker, Dr. Peter Grinspoon."

I started speaking, and it felt entirely comfortable to be up there, opening myself up. As I was launching into my story, I marveled at the fact that, at this very moment, I had come around full circle. I had come from the despair of snorting Oxycontin alone in my office, without any hope, or hope of hope in the future, sick as could be, breaking the law, and harming the very patients I was entrusted to care for. And now I was speaking at this gathering of professionals, who were intently listening to me tell how I had overcome all of this, and how I was able to reinfuse color and joy into my gray and broken life.

Soon after this speech, I was hired by Society to Help Physicians as one of their associate directors, to help assess and monitor physicians with substance abuse disorders. I now sat on the other side of the exact same table and listened patiently to their evasions and to their despair. I see myself in them, an earlier me, grappling with the shambles they have made of their lives, dodging the medical board and the law, sacrificing their families, and everything else, for the next fix. I counsel them, "If you just stop doing drugs, everything is going to work out."

Afterword:
The Addicted Physician

For most of the early part of my medical career, I was the equivalent of a street addict who happened to be wearing a monogrammed lab coat and a stethoscope. I had a prescription pad in my pocket, and I was invested with the responsibility and trust that go along with being a physician. The damage I could have caused is unfathomable.

As physicians, we face unique stressors and access that can predispose us to addiction. We commonly become addicted, at least as often as the rest of the population. We have an estimated 10 to 15 percent lifetime risk of addiction to drugs or alcohol, which is higher than the estimated 9 percent in the general population.

When we do become addicted, we face a colossal stigma that serves as an often-insurmountable barrier to care. Struggling physicians are afraid to seek help, and suffer silently until they self-destruct. The help we are offered is often more punitive than rehabilitative.

The media coverage of physicians in distress tends to be lurid and derisive. We are held to impossibly high standards, and then we fall. When we do fall, we are shunted to the side, sanctioned, stripped of our qualifications, derided, and often deprived of the chance to be healed and to return to a productive life of caregiving. We end up saddled with, and scarred by, guilt and shame.

Ironically, physicians who suffer from addiction tend to do very well, and have success rates that have been quoted as high as 70 to 80 percent. For addiction, this is astronomical. We do well because we have resources to expend on treatment, and we have a lot to fight for.

Doctors in recovery tend to be outstanding doctors who are humble, who listen, and who empathize. Our struggles and our recovery strengthen precisely the qualities that most people seek in a caregiver: compassion and a fine-tuned perception of human vulnerability.

In order to address the problem of addicted physicians, it is critical to understand and address what is causing the current epidemic of physician burnout. We must destigmatize addiction and offer earlier, nonpunitive avenues for individuals to receive help without fear.

Doctors are as ill prepared to deal with death, disease, divorce, or addiction as is the rest of the population. We are thought of as invulnerable, and as not having the same problems that our patients come to see us about. It doesn't help that society sets a standard where doctors aren't supposed to get sick, sad, or tired. Never, during our training, are we encouraged to ask for help in personal matters.

Current medical training, both for students and for residents, has to help educate young doctors about physician health, and has to provide nonthreatening resources if they start to encounter difficulties. We have to equip young doctors with the tools they need to navigate the emotional ups and downs they are going to face in practice life, and the phenomenal stress and temptations that come with being a practicing physician.

The sheer hubris of being a doctor made it easier for me to be in denial about my addiction. I'm at Haaarrvard, aren't I? How drugged-out can I be? If I were really on drugs, I wouldn't have these patients lining up outside my office day after day, waiting for a precious few minutes of my time.

My therapist Ben did his best to burst my bubble. He insisted that I was no different from any of the drug addicts I've cared for, such as those at Boston City, who would disappear just after we put IVs in, and come back high as a kite several hours later, saying, in effect, thanks for the intravenous access.

I couldn't conceive that I had anything in common with these people. Having the cloak of being a physician contributed to this, and allowed me to delay and delay my treatment for years, until I had countless brushes with overdose, and until the state police showed up at my office.

Another dangerous component was that I had unlimited access to pills. Between the samples in the office, the unused medications brought in by patients, the medicines my colleagues would prescribe as "professional courtesy," and the use of my prescription pad, there was no limit to my ability to procure pills. When I called my primary care doctor for Vicodin because of "migraines," he tended to believe me. If a different patient had called, he might have seen through it. It is truly a wonder that I survived at all.

Doctors are also afraid of getting in trouble, which is what can happen, quickly, when you mention to another doctor that you are using drugs or having problems with alcohol. Why would any individual physician ask for help if they knew it could ruin their career?

In a survey published in *JAMA* (the *Journal of the American Medical Association*) in July 2010, 17 percent of physicians reported having had direct personal knowledge of an impaired or incompetent physician in their hospital, group, or practice. Of those, one-third didn't report the individual. Those who kept silent said that they believed someone else was taking care of the problem, they feared retribution, or they worried that the physician would be severely punished.

These statistics are amazing, given that we are "mandated reporters" to the medical board, and that it violates the law to not report an impaired physician.

Docs don't tell on one another in part because the medical board, at least in Massachusetts, can be mercurial, irrational, and punitive. We don't want to take away a colleague's livelihood, or subject them to a Kafkaesque bureaucracy that may never let go of them.

Being an addicted physician, I had the potential to harm many more people than most addicts, though airline pilots and nurses can do a pretty good job. I was the wolf in sheep's clothing. I was deceiving people left and right who trusted me to help them, to "do no harm," and who trusted the establishment I represented.

I had trust and I had power. I had the trust of my patients, the DEA, the medical board, and my colleagues. Everyone gives the doctor the benefit of the doubt. People in other circumstances might have noticed some missing pills, but it never would have occurred to them that *their doctor* was skimming them off the top.

Once I violated my doctorly trust, all hell broke loose. I damaged myself and my profession.

As a physician, the treatment I received was of much higher quality than what almost all other addicts have access to. Most addicts don't have a Society to Help Physicians to force them to abstain. They can't afford rehab, and don't have anything as tangible as a medical license to fight for. I look at the help I received, compared to the substandard care I was exposed to in Maria's dungeon, and can only marvel at those who have brought themselves into recovery without my advantages.

However, my addiction should never have progressed to the point that the state police and the DEA came to my office. This represents a failure, though it's difficult to pinpoint exactly where the failure occurred. If we aren't adequately and compassionately caring for our caregivers, and helping our doctors who are in trouble, and teaching them how to avoid trouble in the first place, then something very fundamental is wrong with our entire system.

Acknowledgments

I acknowledge my caregivers and my friends in the recovery community who helped make my recovery possible. Without them, and without Physician Health Services, I wouldn't have been able to complete this book, or return to medicine.

I would like to acknowledge my family for their support, and their infinite patience with me. My wife, Liz, couldn't possibly have been more supportive in every conceivable way that is possible for a person to be supportive. She read this text so many times that she probably wanted to hang herself. My brother David read drafts all along, encouraged me, and provided critical insights. He helped me navigate the mysterious, byzantine world of publishing as a first-time author. Thank you to my twin brother, Joshua, for sharing memories, for his tremendous support, and for his edits, even if they were terrible and demonstrated a profound misunderstanding of written language. Thank you to my teenage children, Emma, Zach, and Jacob, for supporting or, actually, bearing with me, during the intensive, cyclical process of writing and editing. Thank you to both of my parents, Betsy and Lester Grinspoon, who have always freely encouraged me to read and to write, and who kept our house stocked with great books. Thank you to my unbelievably generous uncle Harold Grinspoon for his support of my recovery.

I would like to acknowledge Dr. Dean Xerras, Dr. Skip Atkins, and Dr. Laura Kehoe, as well as Sheila Arsenault and the rest of the staff at the Chelsea MGH health center for their ongoing support.

I owe a huge thank-you to my agent, Christy Fletcher, for believing in me as an unknown nobody, and for her critical, creative insights along the way, including coming up with the title *Free Refills*. Thank you to Sylvie Greenberg for her phenomenal edits. I wish to thank my editor, Stacy Creamer, for her expert and insightful editing, wonderful ideas, support, and patience with all of my clueless missteps as a first-time author. I wish to acknowledge and thank the staff at Hachette Books, who were welcoming to me, supportive, and profoundly competent from beginning to end, including, but not limited to, Michelle Aielli, Betsy Hulsebosch, Mauro DiPreta, Melanie Gold, and Lauren Hummel.

I wish to acknowledge my close friend Freddy Hackney for being such a great person, and for somehow getting me through rehab. I wish to thank my cousin Ezra Hausman for reading and commenting on the manuscript, and for being my literal and figurative tennis partner. Thank you to Jayne Yaffe Kemp for reading the manuscript and for providing unbelievably good edits.

Finally, I wish to acknowledge my distinguished canine, Benji, despite the fact that he constantly interrupted my work in his endless, existential quest for tummy rubs.